Praise for David Kahn

"David Kahn was able to significantly improve the team members' force protection posture and lethality in the event of a life-threatening altercation. The training provided was a highly valuable complement to the team members' preexisting abilities, as all [members] were able to develop and improve their skills in defense against unarmed attackers, attackers armed with knives or firearms, multiple attackers, and vehicular abduction tactics. Not only did David and Poodie have a wealth of knowledge applicable to a wide variety of unarmed combat scenarios; it was clear that they are continuously doing research and staying informed about emerging threats to US service members in the contemporary operating environment, studying trends and TTPs among potential adversary groups, and developing ways to counter these constantly evolving threats, within the framework of the krav maga system. I would highly recommend continuous future training programs with the IKMA (Gidon system) for all US service members deploying overseas as well as law enforcement officers working domestically in any environment in which they are exposed to the threat of violence."

—**Joshua W. Curtis**, MSG, RIARNG, United States Army 19th Special
Forces Group Operations NCO

"On behalf of the 308 RQS and the USAF SERE community, I would like to thank you [David Kahn]. Your ability to instruct practical self-defense tactics and portray true hand-to-hand combat violence of action in realistic scenarios is one of the best I have seen. Your military-specific 'lethality' training is qualitatively unique and different from any other courses we have attended. I hope and look forward to working with you in the future, not only to improve my knowledge of combatives, but also to improve the whole Air Force Special Operations community!"

—**Michael D. McCune**, SSgt, SERE specialist, USAF

"Bottom line up front. David Kahn and his team are, by far, the best there is, and they teach the best version of the system there is. If you want to arm yourself with the best tools to survive any encounter (civilian, law enforcement, or military combat), David Kahn and the IKMA Gidon system are your best options. I always shop around for the best instructor with the most practical training. David and his team are undeniably the best. There are several different interpretations of krav maga systems available in the United States. Most of them teach substandard techniques. While krav maga is designed to be simple to understand, there still needs to be much emphasis on the subtle, finer points that make a technique effective. David's books are extremely well articulated and spell out every detail of what you need to know from a strategic approach, including all the subtle nuances that make a technique work."

—**Ronald D. Groves**, SFC, United States Army military police lead
instructor, Law Enforcement Training Seminar (LETS)

"David Kahn's krav maga is fighting: brutal, flesh on flesh, and bone on bone. The counter-moves and techniques will take you to an elite level."

—**Aaron Donald**, 2017 and 2018 NFL Defensive Player of the Year, defensive tackle for the Los Angeles Rams

"David Kahn's krav maga gives [me] the ability to break the will of the guy across from me. That is what I'm all about and this [krav maga] will help you do just that!"

—**Khalil Mack**, 2016 NFL Defensive Player of the Year, NFL outside linebacker for the Chicago Bears

"This is the most brutal and violent hand fighting I've learned yet. David Kahn's krav maga is the secret weapon."

—**BJ Finney**, NFL center for the Pittsburgh Steelers

"Israeli krav maga has helped me in a tremendous way to keep defenders off of me. David Kahn's techniques are designed for real combative fighting, but these techniques really help me on the field."

—**Chris Hubbard**, NFL tackle for the Cleveland Browns

"The Krav Maga for Law Enforcement was just remarkable. You and your staff were very attentive to details and knew exactly what our department was looking for. Our instructors had so much good feedback to give. Almost all of the officers agreed that more officers on the street need training like this, and they were eager to engage in any additional training like this that we could provide them. I will definitely continue to use the tactics and techniques taught in your course in teaching officers in-service and recruits. I highly recommend your course to any law enforcement agency or organization that is willing to update their training and give their officers the tools they need to protect themselves in use-of-force situations."

—**Lieutenant Jose Medina**, Philadelphia Police Department, Recruit Training Unit and Reality Based Training Section

"When recommended by the Department of Justice to update our department's use of force training, I kept the fact in mind that suspects are training more and using tactics and techniques taught in mixed martial arts, cage fighting, and ground fighting against officers. I researched several options and found that not all krav maga courses are the same. The term is widely used and the concepts distorted. Mr. Kahn's background as a lawyer has given him a legal perspective. Mr. Kahn has created a law enforcement krav maga course that supports the fundamental tactics that are easy to learn, easy to use, and easy to teach, using instinctive, reflexive body movements. Mr. Kahn was then able to elevate that philosophy as he developed a system that builds on a solid foundation of defensive tactics, giving the officers options when dealing with different types of attacks. Any law enforcement personnel that is forced to face these types of attacks will be better prepared to prevail in those situations by using force options that are appropriate and reasonable if trained properly. Mr. Kahn has given officers the necessary tools needed to properly defend themselves against this new form of street fighting."

—**Sgt. Alfredo Lopez**, Philadelphia Police Department, Philadelphia Police Academy Physical Training and Defensive Tactics Section

"After training with David for ten years, I now have students of my own. I have become even more dependent on David's teachings. My students have varied self-defense backgrounds but marvel at the expedience and efficiency of krav maga."

—**David Rahn**, US Army (retired)

"David Kahn masterfully demonstrates the effectiveness of Israeli krav maga in his outstanding book *Krav Maga Combatives: Maximum Effect*. Kahn's book is well written, thoroughly researched, and is filled with numerous detailed photographs. Early on in a great section, his book expertly delves into the various legal ramifications of self-defense. The major focus of his book is on the practical and valuable selection of basic, intermediate, and advanced bodily weapons or combatives you can use against your opponent. His book describes in depth the combatives to use in self-defense, optimal areas to target on your opponent, and, most importantly, how to properly apply these combatives to achieve maximum effect. I like how he illustrates that Israeli krav maga capitalizes on the whole body for an array of devastating combative options, from upper-body and lower-body striking to grappling. I highly recommend this book for those who want to enhance their survival skills in self-defense situations."

—**Andrew Zerling**, martial arts veteran, multi-award winning author of *Sumo for Mixed Martial Arts*

"David Kahn is a prolific author of books and videos on the Israeli art of krav maga, and his newest book, *Krav Maga Combatives: Maximum Effect*, is not only a supplement and complement to his previous krav maga books and video instructional materials but also an excellent standalone volume that distills krav maga's core combatives into easily digested and understood principles and techniques, and then explains how to apply them for maximum combative effect when forced to physically defend oneself.

"The unique teaching in this volume, that sets this book apart from many martial art books, is the foundation of principles, especially that of attacking an opponent as fast and hard as one can, in the most effective manner possible, while utilizing a continuous attack principle called retzev (or continuous combat motion). He not only illustrates and teaches principles along with effective combative techniques, but he also shows how to combine them in a continuous attack in order to be most effective.

"For any student of krav maga, combatives, or self-defense, this text deserves to be studied and applied to your training to obtain maximum effect when it comes to counterattacking and neutralizing physical threats against you or those you must protect."
—**Alain Burrese, JD**, author, 5th dan Hapkido, former army sniper

KRAV MAGA COMBATIVES

MAXIMUM EFFECT

BECAUSE NOT ALL KRAV MAGA IS THE SAME® . . .
"IMITATION IS THE SINCEREST FORM OF FLATTERY."
—Charles Caleb Colton

KRAV MAGA COMBATIVES

MAXIMUM EFFECT

BY DAVID KAHN

YMAA Publication Center
Wolfeboro, New Hampshire

YMAA Publication Center, Inc.
Main Office:
PO Box 480
Wolfeboro, New Hampshire 03894
1-800-669-8892 • info@ymaa.com • www.ymaa.com

10 9 8 7 6 5 4 3 2 1

ISBN: 9781594396816(print) • ISBN: 9781594396823 (ebook)

First edition. Copyright ©2019 by David Kahn
Editor: T. G. LaFredo
Proofreader: Doran Hunter
Cover design: Axie Breen
Photos provided by David Kahn unless noted otherwise.
This book is typeset in Adobe Garamond Pro.

Publisher's Cataloging in Publication

Names: Kahn, David, 1972– author.
Title: Krav maga combatives : maximum effect / by David Kahn.
Description: First edition. | Wolfeboro, New Hampshire, USA : YMAA Publication Center, [2019] |
    Includes bibliographical references and index.
Identifiers: ISBN: 9781594396816 (print) | 9781594396823 (ebook) | LCCN: 2019936923
Subjects: LCSH: Krav maga. | Krav maga—Training. | Self-defense. | Self-defense—Training. |
    Hand-to-hand fighting. | Hand-to-hand fighting—Training. | Martial arts—Training. | BISAC:
    SPORTS & RECREATION / Martial Arts & Self-Defense. | SOCIAL SCIENCE / Violence in Society.
Classification: LCC: GV1111 .K254 2019 | DDC: 796.81—dc23

Printed in Canada.

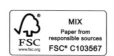

For Claire, Benjamin, and Leo
In loving memory of Helen Brener Smith

An Israeli krav maga blessing
The Book of Psalms, chapter 144:1

לדוד ברוך צורייהוה המלמד לקרבידי אצבעותי למלחמה:

"A Psalm of David. Blessed be the LORD, my rock,
Who trains my hands for war,
And my fingers for battle."

Contents

Foreword: The Krav Maga Combatives Mind-Set

"Better to be a warrior in a garden than a gardener in a war."
—SUN TZU

I decided to start my foreword with a quote from Sun Tzu, one of the greatest minds in history, regarding combat. Since the time of Sun Tzu's writings, to be sure, the art of combat has evolved. As an individual, the need to be prepared to meet today's threats in a volatile world has never been more relevant and prevalent. As a combat veteran, I proudly served in the United States Air Force for over twenty-four years as both an enlisted member and officer. While on active duty, I served alongside some of our nation's most elite, skilled troops, having taken part in missions in pursuit of our nation's high-value tier-1 targets. Hand-to-hand combat was an integral part of our specialized training. I also grew up under some trying circumstances that required me to protect myself from street violence. Accordingly, I gained many reality-based insights about what will work and, equally important, what will not work to defend oneself against both serious social and criminal violence.

Upon retirement from active duty, Israeli krav maga became the focus of my combative studies under David Kahn, chief US instructor for the Israeli Krav Maga Association (Gidon system). With a strong understanding and conviction that "not all krav maga is the same," I have learned an invaluable hand-to-hand combat skill set from David. It has prepared me to face today's violent threats that may confront the everyday citizen. Krav maga was birthed in the violent Middle East by Imi Lichtenfeld. Its teachings still hold true today through the instruction of David Kahn. David's krav maga instruction offers a practical and tactical system to identify, prevent, and, if required, neutralize a threat in a highly efficient and effective manner, using economy of force. This book builds on the foundations set forward by Imi Lichtenfeld and expanded by tenth-dan Grandmaster Haim Gidon, Israeli Krav Maga Association. I wholeheartedly endorse the pages contained within.

Captain (Ret.) Sean P. Hoggs I
US Air Force veteran, Air Force Special Operations command

Acknowledgements

Once more into the breach, I am indebted to Grandmaster Haim Gidon for instilling in his students Israeli krav maga at its supreme professional level. With Imi Lichtenfeld's blessing, Haim continues to advance and improve krav maga as head of the Israeli krav maga system and president of the Israeli Krav Maga Association (Gidon system). Many of the tactics you will see in this book are courtesy of Grandmaster Gidon's unique understanding of what krav maga must be—and, equally important, with all of the different krav maga interpretations now, what it should not be. I always come back from Grandmaster Gidon's gym, located in Netanya, Israel, grateful and indebted for the unequaled training he provides.

Black-belt instructor Rinaldo Rossi and senior instructors Don Melnick and Chris Eckel are instrumental in the development of our instructional materials. Supporting Grandmaster Haim Gidon, the highest-ranking Israeli krav maga instructors are sixth dan Ohad Gidon along with fifth dans Yoav Krayn, Noam Gidon, Yigal Arbiv, Steve Moishe, and Aldema Zirinksi. These individuals represent the epitome of krav maga professional instruction. Aldema is a great friend who has provided immeasurable support and counsel over many years. You will not meet a better, more professionally prepared group of Israeli hand-to-hand combat fighters and instructors.

I am grateful to my great friends Major HC "Sparky" Bollinger, a former Cobra gunship pilot, and Ret. M.Sgt. Ronald E. Jacobs, former chief instructor for the United States Marine Corps Martial Arts Program, who have added to our krav maga abilities and knowledge with their invaluable feedback. We owe great thanks to Capt. (Ret.) Frank Small, who gave us our start in training the United States military. United States Army lead law enforcement M.Sgt. Ronnie Groves is a great supporter and instructor. I am privileged to have Ronnie's support and honored the material is helping our military personnel. The same holds for Army Special Forces M.Sgts. Dan and Josh for their support and professional approval of our training. I am grateful to retired Navy instructors R., J., N., J., and S. and USAF SERE instructors T.Sgts. Mike and Ben for their nonpareil professional insights and support—and, most importantly, for what they all do.

I would like to thank the following additional United States Marine Corps personnel: Lt. Col. Joseph Shusko, Ret.; GySgt. Gokey, Ret.; M.GySgt. Urso, Ret.; and Lt. Col. "Tonto" Ardese, Ret. Thanks also to Sgt. Ben Perkins of the Royal Marines, along with 1st Sgt. Johnson, and Maj. Lanzolloti of the United States Air Force for their support. Maj. Sean Hoggs, Ret., is an amazing supporter of our system and provides invaluable insights into training and life. I am truly honored by Sean's foreword in this book. David Saucier is a great friend and supporter for what we do. "Sauce" is a hero and a survivor.

I must not fail to mention my gratitude to all our fighting men and women of the United States military and Israel Defense Force for safeguarding our freedom.

Sgt. Maj. Nir Maman, Ret., former LOTAR lead counterterror instructor, krav maga instructor, and IDF Infantry and Paratroopers Ground Forces Command Soldier of the Year, 2009, possesses many unequalled professional insights and offers specialized training expertise as only he can provide. Nir has improved the Israeli krav maga system immeasurably. I also have the benefit that Nir is one of my greatest friends. Eyal E. and Dima G. are also great friends and add to our understanding of the Israeli method of defensive measures and close protection. I thank Dr. Neil Farber and Moti Horenstein for inviting me to join the Federation of Israeli Martial Arts' (FIMA) Board of Directors. I am honored to serve as the combatives director for the Israeli Combative Tactics Association (ICTA) arm. I also thank Itay Gil for his kind words.

I am indebted to the Hauerstocks for their *sabra* hospitality in my many visits to Israel and my good friend Shira Orbas, along with her wonderful family. I offer special thanks to Master Kobi Lichtenstein and his organization for their hospitality. Thank you to the IKMA board of directors and all IKMA members, who have welcomed and trained with me over the years. Once again, this book would not be possible without the expert training, support, and inspiration of krav maga's backbone: the IKMA (www .facebook.com/gidonsystemkravmaga/).

Two of the first American krav maga instructors, senior instructors Rick Blitstein and Alan Feldman, are redoubts of support and special reservoirs of krav maga knowledge. I am forever grateful to Rick for sending me on the correct krav maga path. My first krav maga experience with Rick Blitstein floored me both literally and figuratively. Rick and Grandmaster Haim Gidon continue the tradition of flooring students. Some humble pie, judiciously eaten, is a good thing.

Our good friend in Poland, Kris Sawicki, keeps the IKMA at the forefront in Europe. I am grateful to all our students at our Israeli krav maga United States training centers (www.israelikrav.com). I am indebted to many other friends, supporters, and our network of fellow in-house instructors including Paul Karleen, Jeff Gorman, Frank Colluci, Joe Drew, Jonathan Sabin, Kevin Scozarro, Bill McGuire, John Papp, Mike Delahanty, David Ordini, Alec Goenner, Jason Bleitstein, David Rahn, Al Ackerman, Kelly Arlinghaus, Mimi Rowland, Mike McElvin, Dion Privett, Manny Sosa, Kathryn Badger, Andre Kwon, Darius Davis, Marc Scheneider, Darcy Howlett, Kim Delesoy, Suzanne Dougherty, Ray Lucas, Roy Shields, Ronnie Allen, Alex O'Neil, and Sarah Mantz. Instructor Cory Davis, along with his lovely wife, Sheena, keep krav maga training at its best on our final frontier. We have some wonderful support in Paul Gilbert, Adam Peterson, Devora Lapidot, and ABC star reporter Rick Williams, along with all those instructors in the pipeline.

Paul Karleen warrants additional special thanks for his amazing instructional abilities, patience, and outstanding support. Paul also took some of the best krav maga photographs I'll ever be lucky enough to have. Many appear in this book.

Officer Al "Poodie" Carson is family to me and has helped me to change the way NFL players approach the "hands" game. I am grateful to All-Pro NFL players Aaron Donald (2017 Defensive Player of the Year) and Khalil Mack (2016 Defensive Player of the Year)—two of the toughest, most dedicated, and most athletic men one could know. We're grateful to the NFL Jacksonville Jaguars organization for their hospitality, especially head strength coach Tom Myslinski and assistant strength coach and Wounded Warrior Sean Karpf. Thank you to the Jaguars' outstanding players, including Lerentee McCray, who brought us into the organization. We are also grateful to the New York Giants organization, including Pro Bowler Olivier Vernon and Coach Aaron Wellman, for their interest in our training and hospitality. I am also grateful to NFL players Chris Hubbard and BJ Finney for their wonderful support. My law-school friend NFL agent David Canter is appreciated for his support and professional insights. I would also like to thank Princeton University's Charles W. Caldwell Jr. '25 and Head Coach of Football Bob Surace, along with Coach Verbit and the rest of the coaching staff for their interest and support in our Football Combatives Training. We are also grateful to Coach Peterson for his support and generating additional college and NFL interest. Dewayne Brown is a highly appreciated member of our team and a truly amazing conditioning coach.

Justice Mitchell truly does "justice" to our approach and method as only he can, along with Justina Pratt. They are great friends and the best marketers I'll ever know. Justice is a true kravist on the mat and in cyberspace. Sorat and Alexander "Lex" Tungkasiri are family to us in no uncertain terms. My son Benjamin, along with his best pal "Lex" and my other son Leo, all budding kravists, beat me up as they should.

Instructor Enrique Prado deserves big thanks for his support. I am also grateful to Kim and Oliver Pimley for their dedication. As ever, the Tenenbaums and Goldbergs remain pillars of my life and *mishpachat*. Paul Szyarto, one tough dude, deserves a superlative thanks for his support and vision. The Graham family is a great bastion of support, especially our mustachioed brawler, "Action Jackson."

Photographer Brandon Jones (www.truestill.studio) did a superb job, and his amazing professionalism and skills helped make this book what it is.

Special thanks on both a personal and professional level to all our friends and supporters in the law enforcement community, including Det. Gioscio; Director Masseroni; Col. Britcher; Lt. Miller, Ret.; Sgt. McComb, Ret.; Sgt. Klem, Ret.; Sgt. Oehlmann; Sgt. Rayhon; Sgt. Ashkar; Lt. Critelli; Sgt. Maniace; Maj. Ponenti; Lt. DeMaise; Lt. Wolf; Lt. Cowan; Sgt. Boland; Chief Trucillo; Capt. Capriglione; Lt. Miano; Lt. Peins; Officer Vaval; Officer Vacirca; Capt. Maimone, Ret.; Lt. Cowan; Corp. Barr; Capt. Savalli, Ret.; Director Harrison; Chief Lazzarotti, Ret.; Director Paglione, Ret.; Lt. Colon; Sgt. Hayden, Ret.; Officer Johnson; Special Agent-in-Charge Hammond; Special Agents Schroeder and Belle; Special Agents Love, Clark, and Baucom; Special Agent Crowe; Captain Laskiewicz; Sheriff Smith; Sheriff Kemler, Chief Warrant Officer Amantia, and the entire Mercer County Sheriff's Office; Commissioner Ross; Chief Werner;

Lt. Medina; Officer Hobson; Sgt. Lopez; Lt. Jose Medina; Sgt. Gill; Sgt. Fitzgerald; Lt Watson; Lt. Rabinovitz; Officer Hosgood; Chief Sutter; Lt. Maurer, Officer Heath, and my entire hometown Princeton Police Department; along with the many other law enforcement professionals with whom we have the honor of working.

Security expert Steven Hartov, one of my favorite authors and good friends, deserves much gratitude for his personal and professional support. I am grateful to Drs. Steven Gecha, Stephen Hunt, and Bruce Rose, as well as PTs Kristin Williams, Lindsay Balint, and Jeff Manheimer for continuing to hold me together. Thanks to Jerry Palmieri for his all-pro conditioning advice, along with Autumn Magee and "Doc" Mark Cheng. I also know I am always in good hands literally and figuratively with my kravist counselor-at-law David Schroth. I thank him for his legal prowess and support.

My family as always is my foundation, especially my wife Claire, mother Anne, and father Alfred, for the growth of krav maga training and all the effort that has gone into expanding our support group. Benjamin and Leo are the next generation of kravists. I hope my sons, like all our students, will be gentlemen with ungentlemanly self-defense capabilities, should the need arise. If I had daughters, I'd want them to be ladies capable of unladylike violence.

Introduction

We are proud to present *Krav Maga Combatives: Maximum Effect.* Once again, we thank the many readers and krav maga enthusiasts who have contacted us about a latest book in the line. This book is designed to both supplement and complement our previous krav maga books and video instructional materials. The goal is to explain and depict krav maga's core combatives—to show how to apply them for maximum combative effect within the legal parameters of self-defense.

In this sixth book we continue to expand the reader's self-defense fighting arsenal based on Israeli krav maga's core combatives as taught by Grandmaster Haim Gidon. This book is designed for a legally responsible person to use optimized combatives to improve his or her chances of surviving an unarmed or armed attack without sustaining serious injury. These combatives stem from my translation of technique guidelines from the Israeli Krav Maga Association (Gidon system).

An irrefutable fact is that one need only learn a few combatives to be an effective fighter. Simple is easy. Easy is effective. Effective is what is required to end a violent encounter quickly and decisively on your terms. For self-defense and fighting purposes, a universally well-known fundamental principle is to attack an opponent as fast and as hard as one can.

But aggression, speed, and force aren't necessarily enough. *How* you use your combatives is crucial. Particularly salient for krav maga self-defense is the observation by the great physicist Albert Einstein: "If you don't have time to do it right, when will you have time to do it over?" In other words, if you don't stop an attacker in the first instance, you may not have the time or opportunity to incapacitate him before he does egregious harm to you. This book stresses doing the right things and doing them in the right way. You may not have another chance. The simple maxim applies: do it right the first time.

Whenever I return from Israel, I come home with a solemn respect for avoiding unnecessary violence at all costs. By unnecessary violence, I mean any confrontational situation we can walk away from without having to physically preempt or use counter-violence. I emphasize this point for two reasons. First, the only fight you are sure to win is one you avoid. Second, paradoxically, I am naturally repelled by the level of violence our krav maga is designed to wreak in a matter of seconds. I have no desire to maim another person unless that person is determined to inflict egregious bodily harm and cannot be deterred otherwise.

Good tactical minds often think alike. Whatever your martial arts or defensive tactics background—or if you have none at all—my hope is that the following material can add some additional defensive combatives and combinations to your repertoire. In addition, with diligent work, this book, especially when combined with our video materials (www.masteringkravmaga.com), will infuse a basic understanding of retzev, continuous combat motion unique to Grandmaster Gidon's krav maga instruction. When facing a potentially deadly situation with no escape, retzev provides no quarter to incapacitate a dangerous, determined, and violent adversary. Proper retzev nearly eliminates an opponent's ability to counter or escape your counterviolent onslaught. We will describe retzev in greater detail later in this chapter and illustrate it in the combatives chapters.

Our aim is to augment your capabilities—to add additional arrows to your quiver. Accordingly, our aim is also to help your aim. In the interest of providing a concise approach, I have tried to include summarizations of a few essential combative-related topics from my previous books, specifically, *Krav Maga* (2004) and *Advanced Krav Maga* (2008). In addition to new photos shot for this book, we have also interspersed a few photos we used previously. This is to further illustrate key combatives in action. These are taken from my books *Krav Maga Professional Tactics* (2016) and *Krav Maga Defense* (2016).

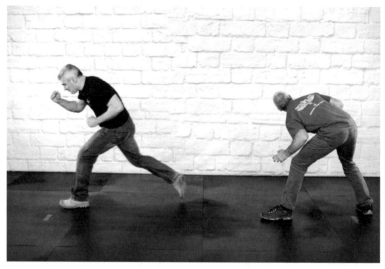

Escape by running away.

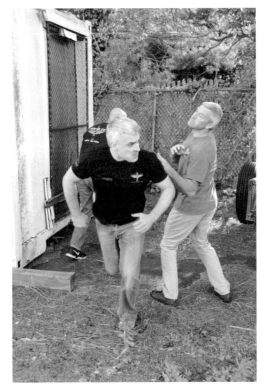

Escape by running away.

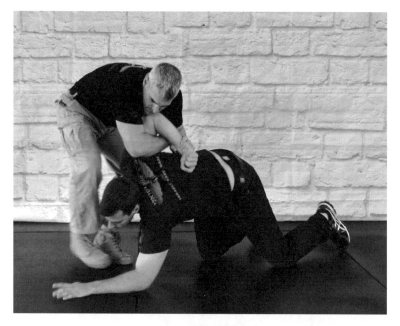

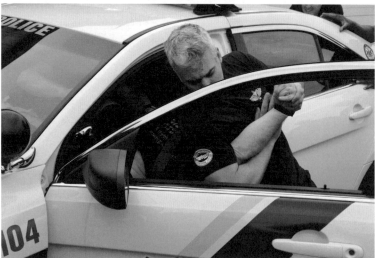

Police restraint and control holds.

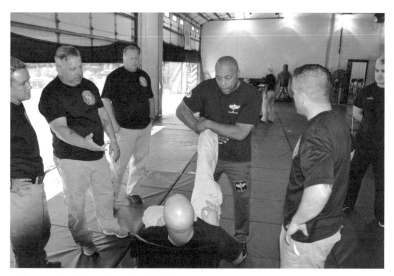

Police restraint and control holds.

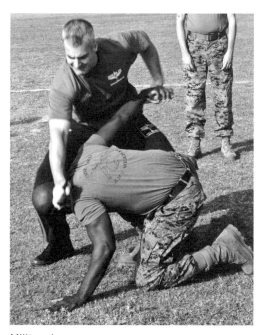

Military krav maga.

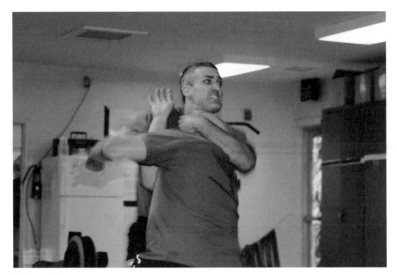

Military krav maga.

This book draws on materials from the first three belt levels of the Israeli krav maga curriculum (yellow, orange, and green). Our goal in training civilians, law enforcement, and military personnel is the same: to deliver a person from harm's way. Civilian krav maga focuses on avoiding, deescalating, escaping, and, if necessary, incapacitating an attacker. Police Krav Maga™ focuses on restraint and control. Military Krav Maga™ focuses on lethal-force applications. There is a definite overlap among civilian, law enforcement, and military training. The crucial differences lie in civilian liability, use-of-force guidelines, and rules-of-engagement considerations. The various photos in this section portray training situations and the goals for all three groups: (1) a civilian disengaging after felling an assailant and running away, (2) law enforcement holds for arrest and control, and (3) military lethal-force applications.

As the highest-ranking krav maga instructor in the world, Grandmaster Haim Gidon continues to evolve and improve the defensive system. I firmly believe krav maga founder Imi Lichtenfeld appointed Haim as Imi's successor to steward krav maga's future progress. In my opinion, many of the improvements and additions you will see in this book are examples of this advancement. Imi knew Haim would do it, and, to be sure, Haim has.

What is paramount is that we do not approach our specific Israeli krav maga training as an exercise program or fad. Unfortunately, the krav maga system is becoming widely known as a workout craze or wildly aggressive, poorly executed, ineffective self-defense. These combatives do indeed provide a superb workout when practiced against a heavy bag, with a partner holding pads, while facing a mirror and practicing solo, or under controlled sparring conditions. But they must be executed properly for both effectiveness in a real situation and for safety in training.

We do not just make up tactics for the sake of being different or putting a personal spin on our training in an attempt to sell it to the public. The tactics and strategies we teach are designed *by* and *for* no-nonsense, tactically minded people who are serious about safety training. These tactics must be effective when confronting a serious threat—someone who will not back down or stop until you stop him.

For those who convert these proven tactics and strategies for their own use without attribution, you know who you are. We know who you are. **Because not all krav maga is the same®.**

The Language of Krav Maga Combatives

Throughout *Krav Maga Combatives* the following terms will appear frequently. Once you understand the language of krav maga, you can better understand the method.

360 outside defense: A series of arm movements coupled with outside rotations to intercept and block an outside attack such as a hook punch.

Cavalier: A wrist takedown forcing an adversary's wrist to move against its natural range of motion, usually combined with *tai sabaki* (defined below) for added power.

Combative: Any manner of strike, takedown, throw, joint lock, choke, or other offensive fighting movement.

Deadside: The position behind an adversary. When you are to the rear of your adversary and your adversary cannot use both arms and legs against you, you are facing his or her deadside.

De-escalation stance: A posture where you have your hands up at chest level and your palms facing a potential adversary.

Fight timing: Using the appropriate tactic at the correct time.

Glicha: A sliding movement on the balls of your feet to carry your entire body weight forward and through a combative strike to maximize its impact. To maximize moving your body weight through the combative strike, move on the balls of your feet forward toward the opponent. The movement of each foot is more of a slide than a step. The lead foot initiates as the rear foot seamlessly follows. The sliding steps with both feet are best kept equidistant to ensure a solid base to complete the combative strike and facilitate additional combatives as necessary (retzev).

Gunt: Angled elbow block defense.

Kravist: A term I coined in 2004 to describe a smart and prepared krav maga fighter.

Left outlet stance: A fighting stance with the left leg forward.

Liveside: The position in front of an adversary. When you are in front of your adversary and your adversary can see you and use both arms and legs against you, you are facing his or her liveside.

Nearside: The side of your adversary closest to your torso. For example, if your adversary's left arm is the limb closest to you, that is his nearside limb.

Off the line: A position that is to the left or right of the trajectory of an actual or anticipated attack. "Move off the line" or "move offline" means to reposition the body to one side or another.

Passive stance: A "negative five" posture where you are unprepared for conflict. You are standing flat-footed and not bladed, paying attention to something other than a threat.

Personal weapons: Hands, feet, body limbs, head, and teeth.

Retzev: A Hebrew word that means "continuous." It is used in krav maga to describe "continuous combat motion." The backbone of modern Israeli krav maga, retzev teaches you to move your body instinctively in combat motion without thinking about your next move. When in a dangerous situation, you'll automatically call upon your physical and mental training to launch a seamless, overwhelming counterattack, using strikes, takedowns, throws, joint locks, chokes, or other offensive actions, combined with evasive action. Retzev is quick and decisive movement merging all aspects of your krav maga training. Defensive movements transition automatically into offensive movements to neutralize the attack, affording your adversary little time to react. Retzev is a force multiplier, increasing the effectiveness of your defense.

Right outlet stance: A fighting stance with the right leg forward.

Secoul: A larger step than glicha, covering more distance to carry your entire body weight forward and through a combative strike to maximize its impact.

Sliding stabbing defense: A defensive arm motion from a resting position of your arm at your side. Project your arm at approximately a 45-degree angle with your fingers held tightly together and the slightest bend in both the wrist and elbow. This is to intercept an incoming attack by deflecting and sliding the attack down your arm.

Tai sabaki: A step of 180 degrees or a shorter range, initiated by either leg and used to about-face. Tai sabaki is used in both defensive footwork, to move the body away from an attack, and offensively, to take down an opponent.

Trapping: Pinning or grabbing the adversary's arms with one arm, leaving you free to continue combatives with your other arm.

The Optimum Use of This Book

Practice each tactic in order as presented. The Israeli krav maga system relies on a few core self-defense combatives adaptable to most violent encounters. Obviously, no book is a substitute for hands-on learning with a qualified Israeli krav maga instructor (please visit www.israelikrav.com). Our overarching goal is to impart some of krav maga's key combatives to sharpen your self-defense skills in the specific situations we cover and, by extension, other related situations. Be sure to thoroughly vet any instructor with whom you should decide to train.

CHAPTER 1

Not All Krav Maga Is the Same

Krav Maga's Critics

I am concerned for the future of krav maga. Imi Lichtenfeld created too formidable a fighting method for it to be relegated to the pile of self-defense and exercise fads. Grandmaster Haim Gidon has spent fifty years enhancing Imi's teachings and producing several generations of instructors who have both become and helped train some of Israel's most capable and finest warriors. I have included the following section to help explain why krav maga has become a bit of a joke within varied professional training circles, underscoring the need for the system to be taught correctly to reestablish its once-stellar reputation.

With krav maga's rapid commercialization and the spread of McDojos offering krav maga, the US military and law enforcement communities now understandably view krav maga somewhat skeptically. Krav maga is also increasingly disparaged in varying degrees by professional mixed martial arts (MMA) fighters. Fortunately, we are able to work with many military units and law enforcement agencies, as well as serious fighters. We help them improve their skill sets and disabuse their preconceived ideas about krav maga's inefficacy. However, we are fighting an uphill battle, as I will explain.

I am not attempting to use this book to grandstand and say splinter krav maga interpretations of Israeli fighting styles are no good. The history of krav maga's efficacy and its (im)proper dissemination will be the arbiter of what is and is not legitimate krav maga. The tragedy is that some lives may be lost, along with people sustaining serious injuries because many current charlatan krav maga instructors do not understand what tactics work in real situations. In other words, while many of these dubious instructors may be well intentioned, they don't grasp that poorly conceived, untested tactics can get you severely injured or killed in short order.

Many people lay claim to being genuine—teaching and making statements they say are true to the system. And yet, much of the material being peddled is suspect according to the IKMA curriculum and often undermines or contradicts Imi's teaching and philosophies. In short, their teaching practices are questionable. More and more unqualified instructors are creating their own "krav maga" systems. Some of them sell krav maga belt rankings at all levels for anyone willing to pay, including degrees and belts available for purchase on the internet. No wonder krav maga is receiving negative reviews—and deservedly so. As krav maga becomes increasingly popular, we suspect that the Israeli fighting system's reputation and efficacy will continue to decline internationally.

The IKMA is the original governing body for Israeli krav maga, recognized by the Israeli government and headed by Grandmaster Haim Gidon. In June 1996, Haim Gidon received his eighth dan (black belt), when krav maga founder Imi Lichtenfeld also declared that ninth and tenth dans (red belt) were to come. The only other instructor to formally receive an eighth dan from Imi was the late Eli Avigzar. Following in Imi's legendary footsteps, after Imi's passing in 1998, Haim became the highest-ranking krav maga instructor in the world.

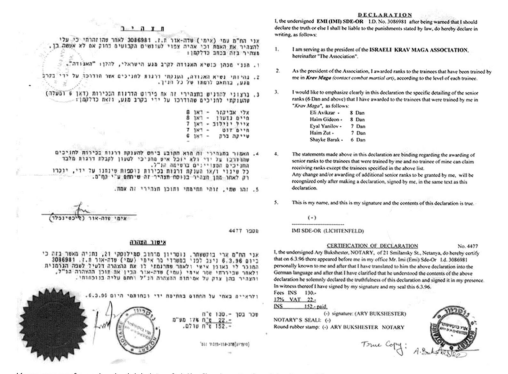

Krav maga founder Imi Lichtenfeld's final notarized belt rankings.

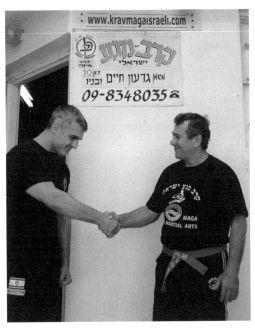

The author with Grandmaster Haim Gidon (Netanya, Israel, 2010).

To be sure, the top-ranked Israeli instructors listed in Imi's final belt-ranking declaration are all highly qualified—as is a select cadre of other instructors not listed who were also awarded black belts by Imi. Any ranked instructor taught by the individuals listed in the above declaration is likely legitimate. As more people become instructors without formal training from Imi's select few top disciples, krav maga's basic core tactics—let alone its more advanced fighting tactics—continue to be ruined and misinterpreted.

Now, people seem to just make up whatever techniques they wish and call them krav maga. Oftentimes, these are complicated and miss the point (and target) altogether. And the public, without the benefit of professional insights, generally cannot distinguish the crucial difference. Some recent popular books and videos underscore a significant lack of understanding of what krav maga was originally intended to be. When instructors claim to have a "broader view" of krav maga and yet violate krav maga's fundamental principles, I view this type of explanation and faulty reasoning as an excuse for what they do not know.

Charles Caleb Colton is often quoted: "Imitation is the sincerest form of flattery." People attempt to copy and replicate what Imi and a select few top instructors do. Some try to do it honorably, others less so. The internet provides an unequaled platform to present claims and, one would hope, an equal opportunity to present indisputable facts to support these claims. We have always operated by the adage that the cream will rise to the top. Unfortunately, savvy marketing churns out spoiled cream rather quickly.

We are acutely aware that popular opinion, over time, can become confused for fact. We believe the krav maga community is entitled to informed opinions and hope to disseminate reliable information. Notwithstanding, this simple truism is correct: people do not know what they do not know. Subpar krav maga may be viewed as competent krav maga because people do not know the difference. While there is more latitude in defending against an unarmed attack, sometimes the all-important subtleties that provide for a successful defense, rather than one that fails and possibly gets you killed, are not recognized. ***Which krav maga approach you follow could be a life-and-death issue.***

Good students ask why. Good instructors explain why. Bad instructors, conversely, brush off such vital questions or respond with "because that's what I learned" as a result of a lack of fundamental knowledge.

The "How" Is Vital

Among the many claimants who say they have the best and most effective krav maga, there are some who assert that krav maga need only provide a skeleton for defensive actions, a set of choices, as it were, that determine what response to use. If a situation calls for a kick, exactly how the kick should be delivered is not so important, and each teacher or practitioner is free to do the kick as he wishes. Or if a punch seems to be the best response to a threat, the exact way to deliver that punch is up for grabs. In other words, beyond calling for the use of feet or fists or elbows or knees, krav maga is represented as eclectic regarding how the response is carried out. I strongly disagree. ***How you carry out a defense is as important as what defense you choose.***

Indeed, there is a correct way to deliver a combative such as a knee, a punch, a palm heel, an elbow, an eye gouge, or a cavalier #1 takedown, along with the best way to bite someone (canting one's head slightly to make maximum use of the incisors). But how should we define "correct"? ***The correct way is the one that is most likely to stop the threat and keep you safe. Shouldn't this be the acid test for the validity of a krav maga response to a threat?***

Claiming the details of techniques are secondary to overarching general principles is really a cover up for an instructor's lack of knowledge when he or she performs a defense incorrectly. Imi Lichtenfeld developed specific movements to optimize the human body's performance. Haim Gidon further optimized these movements while also enhancing and expanding krav maga to contend with modern violent threats. *There is the correct way* (including, on occasion, a few options) to execute Imi's krav maga defense. And then there is every other way.

Finally, many instructors focus purely on the commercial aspects—namely, adding the tag "krav maga" to their schools to capitalize on an industry buzzword. These schools are more focused on the money coming in than the quality of the material going out. If they were serious about teaching legitimate krav maga, they would do their research. They would engage a reputable krav maga organization. As this takes more time and effort than most care to invest, they take the easy path at the expense of their earnest krav maga students.

The paramount point is this: fighting for your life is not a sport. There is no referee. You cannot replay first down. If you must act when faced with a deadly force situation, your life is on the line, and the lives of your family and companions may also hang in the balance.

Everyday Maximum Effect

Here's a principle that can apply everywhere in life:

How you do something is as important
as what you choose to do.

This book stresses both the *how* and the *what* of krav maga: doing the right things in the right way to achieve maximum effect—stopping the threat and doing it safely. We can put this in the form of a simple equation:

Correct Technique + Correct Execution = Maximum Effect

The goal of this book is to help you develop a range of tools, defenses that really get the job done safely and effectively for a maximum effect. We come back to Einstein: "If you don't have time to do it right, when will you have time to do it over?"

Overarching Krav Maga Principles

When evaluating whether a technique and its usage will have maximum effect, it helps to lay out a few immutable krav maga principles. They inform both the choice of a tactic and the way to execute it. If we meet these principles, we would generally deem the approach acceptable and therefore *maximum-effect krav maga*.

Krav Maga's Core Combative Principles

Relying on optimized combatives, krav maga's overarching strategy is to take whatever practical measures are necessary to deliver a defender from harm's way. When situational avoidance, de-escalation, and escape are not possible, Israeli krav maga uses twelve broad self-defense principles:

1. Utilize a preemptive, targeted counterattack against an attacker's anatomical vulnerabilities. When this is not possible, utilize simultaneous or near-simultaneous defense and attack. This includes an instinctive body defense combined with a deflection, block, or redirection of the attack, embedded with the necessary ferocity of counterviolence to thwart the attack.

2. Deliver initial counterattacks that optimize your body's natural, instinctive motions, yielding maximum power and reach. Pivot and use the body's full mass to drive through a combative while allowing for instinctive follow-on combatives. In other words, generate as much speed and power as your physique will allow, using retzev (continuous combat motion).

3. Target the attacker's anatomical vulnerabilities, sequentially, if possible, while facilitating retzev. Bear in mind that you must use only objectively reasonable counterforce. When the attacker is no longer a threat, you must cease your counterattack immediately.

4. Use visceral defensive tactics devoid of any sporting aspect, both when standing and if you are unavoidably forced to the ground.

5. Train tactics that reasonably work for you, keeping in mind that krav maga's objective is to provide practical, instinctive solutions for any defender, regardless of size, strength, or athletic ability.

6. Keep your body and hands properly positioned. Use good footwork, and do not drop your hands. If possible, do not commit both hands to the same movement.

7. Use any type of available improvised weapon (a mobile device, parked vehicle, wall, furniture, magazine, book, or laptop, for example) or designated weapon, where legal to carry one. Beware that during the course of a violent encounter, your assailant may attempt to do the same.

8. Use tactics flexible enough to work against related attack movements or a "family of attacks." For example, the same defensive tactic will work against a hook punch, a hook edged-weapon stab, an overhead edged-weapon stab, and an edged-weapon slash.

9. Train tactics that work against determined, concerted resistance or imme-diate countertactics an attacker might attempt to use. In other words, the tactics must work against an adversary who is trained in martial arts or hand-to-hand combat. This, in part, focuses on proper body mechanics and dead-side positioning.

10. Utilize economy of motion and simplicity without telegraphing your intent or strategy. This applies to the use of personal weapons as well as the ability to incorporate improvised or dedicated weapons.

11. Beware of the tactical environment, including weather conditions (wet ground, ice) and obstacles, such as a curb, parked vehicle, wall, or furniture. Recall that these items may also be used as improvised weapons.

12. Utilize tactics that work against multiple assailants and that position you to the deadside, especially when confronting multiple assailants. Do everything you can to avoid going to the ground or being taken down.

In the following sections you will see combatives that conform to these twelve core principles. In addition, you will be exposed to many technical details showing when and why that particular approach to a defensive situation is effective. Our goal with this book is for you to take good combatives and optimize them in usage, honing them into the most formidable and effective fighting method.

BECAUSE NOT ALL KRAV MAGA IS THE SAME®. . . .

CHAPTER 2

Key Strategies for Achieving Maximum Effect

This section continues the *how* of effective krav maga in terms of key approaches that lead to the best results.

Attacking the Attacker

Israel is a small country approximately the size of the state of New Jersey. Because of its small geographic footprint and dense population centers, the Israeli defensive outlook is to prevent a fight from happening on Israeli soil. Rather, the doctrine of the Israel Defense Force (IDF) is to take the fight to an enemy whenever possible—on his turf. Israeli krav maga is an extension of this doctrine: **attack the attacker**. Do not absorb damage. Instead, violently turn the tables on your attacker, either preemptively or with combined defense and attack.

Krav maga should be translated as "contact combat." Combat is a life-and-death battle bereft of any rules or fight etiquette. The Israeli krav maga self-defense system's combatives are known for brutal efficiency. Importantly, correctly taught krav maga recognizes that the attacker will resist and try to physically overwhelm you without conceding defeat.

Targeted, injurious counterviolence against an attacker leads to a conclusive result: the scale of physical power tilts in the kravist's favor. A few elementary core tactics that can be performed instinctively and adapted to myriad situations will deliver you from harm's way. Knowing how to maim an attacker by striking vital points and organs or applying choking or breaking pressure to an attacker's joints will end the violent encounter decisively and on your terms.

The key is your mind-set: to neutralize an opponent quickly and decisively. Your violent intent or aggression governs your ability to inflict visceral counterviolence. In violent conflict, the party who significantly damages the other party first usually prevails, especially if he or she presses the counterattack home to neutralize the threat. In other words, the victor is whoever first successfully exploits an opponent's anatomical vulnerability with a well-placed debilitating combative—*and* continues to serially injure the opponent through retzev. Survivors do not vacillate in imposing their will on an attacker to alter the outcome.

Preemption

It cannot be emphasized enough that krav maga stresses preemptive tactics. As the kravist, you are provided with an all-important preemption capability prior to the full initiation of an attack. Your goal is to thwart an assailant's freedom of action by recognizing the warning signs of impending violence. Obviously, such early recognition allows for preventing a negative outcome. If avoidance is not possible, then early detection enables preemptive counterviolence to thwart an attack at its inception rather than waiting for it.

For example, if you see an attack coming, depending on the distance, you can launch a kick that stops the aggressor where he is. Isn't it better to keep the attacker away with your legs than to have to engage him with your fists or elbows, where he is closer to you to inflict damage? This kind of maximum-effect approach can stop the aggressor cold and is more likely to keep you safe.

Determining range and distance coupled with timing is paramount to successfully using preemptive linear kicks—and all other combatives. For example, imagine you have properly extended your leg to deliver a kick. While human anatomical proportions differ considerably, for argument's sake, let's consider the length of your extended leg to represent about 50 percent of your height. This is based on iliac height, or the distance between the top of the iliac crest (the top of your hip) and the floor. To perform an effective or optimum kick (straight or side kick) with correct base-leg pivot, the closest distance you can allow someone near you is approximately half your height. This translates to somewhere between two and a half feet for shorter defenders and three and a half feet for the tallest defenders.

Examples:

If you stand about 5′4″ (64 inches), then your minimum linear kick distance must be 32 inches, or about two and a half feet.

If you stand about 5′10″ (70 inches), then your minimum linear kick distance must be 35 inches, or about three feet.

Importantly, when using a base-leg glicha sliding step, you can considerably expand the long-distance range of your preemptive attack. For roundhouse kicks using the shin to strike, the range is approximately the same as that of a linear straight punch. This is why roundhouse kicks combined with straight punches create a natural striking combination.

Fight Timing

Indispensable to a successful defense is correct fight timing, or using an appropriate tactic at the correct time. Preemption and fight timing are a fusion of instinct with simultaneous decision-making.

> **Fight-Timing Essentials**
> - You have the choice to (1) either preempt an opponent's attack by initiating your own attack or (2) react to an opponent's attack by countertargeting a physical vulnerability the opponent exposes.
> - When attacking, even a skilled opponent leaves himself open briefly for counterattack. For example, as the opponent delivers a straight punch or a series of upper-body combatives, he shifts his weight forward, offering you the opportunity to deliver a side kick to the knee, thereby crippling him.

Optimizing Combatives

The old adage singularly applies: the best defense is a superior offense. The IDF relies on quality of military prowess instead of quantity—though, of course, quantity is always welcome. This is especially true when facing multiple adversaries at the same time—another difficult scenario the IDF is often accustomed to seeing. A similar analogy may be made for Israeli krav maga as well. It is a select group of optimized, superior tactics, adaptable to many situations, that brings overwhelming firepower to bear in a time of need. It is crucial to remember krav maga's historical roots. Jewish defenders were usually outnumbered by attackers. Accordingly, Imi Lichtenfeld developed krav maga to fend off multiple attackers. There was precious little time to defeat one attacker before another one pounced. Therefore, each combative had to count; each had to be optimized.

Aggression is a prerequisite for effectively wielding counterviolence. Your mind-set must be to overcome any unavoidable threat that poses a danger. Combine aggression, a no-lose resolve, and optimized combatives to prevail. Regardless of what type of combative strike you deliver, shifting your body weight forward to deliver the strike will allow you to place all your body mass behind it, connecting with greater force. Grandmaster Gidon emphasizes that without the proper execution—optimum execution—of krav maga's essential combatives, there can be no effective krav maga. Again, this is the *what* (choice of combative) plus the *how* (optimum execution). In other words, if you do not learn how to harness your maximum potential to deliver a combative to consequently damage another human being who is determined to harm you, you sell yourself short—which can get you seriously injured or killed. Whatever you weigh, however tall or short you are, and whatever strength you possess must all be single focused into driving your body through an opponent to end the attack.

While a kick to the groin or knee is usually effective, why not maximize the effect? When we train law enforcement and military, we generally do not have significant time to teach a large set of combatives. To achieve a rapid learning curve, we co-opt whatever combatives the trainees already know and simplify the range of tactics. This can also work for civilians. However, *if you have the time to train*, it befits you to learn something to the best of your ability. So, for example, I advocate learning a superior straight kick by turning the base leg—rather than an inferior straight kick with both your feet pointed in the same direction. The base-leg turn for a straight kick provides an optimum linear strike, harnessing one's center mass along the femur to drive the force through the opponent. Pivoting correctly on the anchoring foot also provides greater extension for the striking limb and lessens the chance of knee injury for the anchor. Other examples include the following:

- For a rear straight punch or palm-heel strike, pivot on the ball of the rear foot in your stance.
- For a rear straight kick or knee, pivot on the ball of the foot of your lead base leg.

The following photos show the entry into the knee strike and the subsequent base-leg foot pivot and turn. Note the clear change in alignment of the base-leg foot and the resulting extra extension.

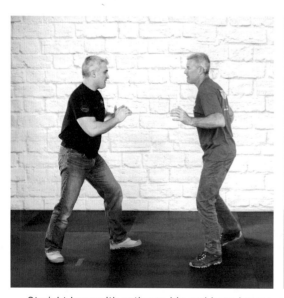 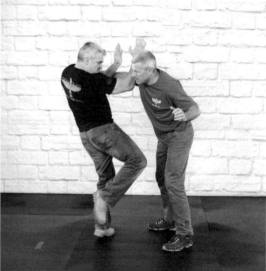

Straight knee with optimum hip and base-leg movement.

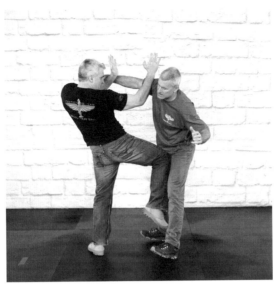

Straight knee with optimum hip and base-leg movement.

Realistic Training

With proper intense training, you can learn effective physical tactics, while mentally adjusting to a simulated, harsh, violent reality. Realistic practice improves reaction capability by allowing an immediate assessment of a violent situation and triggering a corresponding stress-simulated reaction. Here are three key goals of such training:

- To adopt and streamline the krav maga method and personalize the techniques to make them your own. This begins conceptually and ends tactically.

- To practice with different partners to become accustomed to the strengths, capabilities, movements, and approaches of different people.

- To sort out your ballistic strikes and combatives, arriving at the ones you feel most comfortable with and that give you the greatest confidence.

Krav maga's defensive philosophy is never to do more than necessary but to instinctively use violence of action incorporating speed, economy of motion, and the appropriate measure of decisive counterforce. Instinctive trained reactions targeting the attacker's anatomical vulnerabilities reign supreme.

In the basest, most animalistic sense—provided the circumstances are legally justifiable—the kravist, when faced with a life-threatening situation, understands how to inflict terrible, debilitating wounds against an adversary. Wounding an assailant balances power in the kravist's favor. Accordingly, a kravist trains as if compelled to *simulate* breaking bones, disabling ligaments, destroying an eyeball, crushing an adversary's windpipe, maiming, crippling, or killing.

The foundation of the krav maga system's methods and philosophy is the ferocious, optimum use of counterviolence. Within this realistic approach, genuine krav maga takes into account personal limitations that may be imposed on the defender's movements and flexibility or an individual's morphology. Note well that certain combatives used by a lithe, unencumbered martial arts fighter with years of training are likely to be significantly different from techniques available to the average person in a street setting. Hence, for our purposes, all krav maga combatives must be practical for the average person. The krav maga system's pledge—and brilliance—is to teach practical combatives so anyone can successfully mount a defense against a violent assault.

Use-of-Force and Legal Considerations

If avoidance, de-escalation, and escape fail, never waver about resorting to counterviolence in the face of violence. Optimized self-defense focuses not simply on survival, but rather on how to neutralize the aggressor. There is no pity or humanity in a desperate, visceral self-defense situation—provided the counterforce is legally justifiable. Legally, you must be able to articulate what you did and why you did it. Your actions must be objectively reasonable to allow for an affirmative defense, should you face legal inquiry.

Counterattacks, especially using retzev, must be considered and understood within a legal use-of-force context. When there is no choice but to use counterforce against a potential deadly force threat (who cannot be reasoned with or otherwise deterred), you, the kravist, must temporarily incapacitate or, if necessary, maim an attacker. For civilian self-defense, we do not advocate in any way killing an attacker unless it is absolutely necessary and within the scope of a deadly force encounter. To avoid legal ramifications, you must articulate why you injured an attacker.

It behooves us to once again remember how and why krav maga was developed. Of course, the answer is self-defense. However, it was a specific "battle zone" type of self-defense. Imi developed krav maga to contend with threats from hostile fellow civilians in prewar Slovakia, terrorists, and enemy combatants all of whom gave no quarter. Krav maga's founding philosophy and tactics recognized that legal liability and jeopardy were usually inapplicable, if not entirely irrelevant in those particular settings. Visceral counterviolence was generally both warranted and required to survive these situations. There was just one overwhelming rule: survive.

Modern Self-Defense Requirements

Today, when civilians employ self-defense, laws govern the proportionality of permissible counterforce. Self-defense may be defined as reasonably necessary counterforce to protect yourself from suffering potential injury or death. If you use and claim self-defense, you will be scrutinized by the police and, quite possibly, the local prosecutor. They will examine closely if your self-defense actions were justified and objectively reasonable.

Laws vary according to jurisdiction, but generally speaking, verbally threatening an individual is assault, while the unwanted touching or striking of a person is battery. Assault and battery often occur together, which is why the terms are used interchangeably among the public. Increasingly, as well, the terms are also used synonymously in courts of law. The three elements of battery are some iteration of the following:

1. A volitional act
2. Orchestrated to cause a harmful or offensive contact with another person under such circumstances that make contact substantially certain to occur
3. Resulting in nonconsensual contact

In the United States, a physical attack (or even the threat of an attack) is usually classified as an assault, a battery, or both. The modern trend is to classify a physical attack as a type of assault. Some states alternatively define assault as an intentional act precipitating fear of imminent bodily harm inflicted by another person. As noted, increasingly, modern statutes do not distinguish between the crime of battery and assault. In other words, statutes often refer to crimes of physical violence as assaults.

Depending on the gravity of the attack, including whether a weapon was used, an assault can be elevated to a level of aggravated assault. To convict a person of assault (or battery in some states), a prosecutor must prove beyond a reasonable doubt that the crime included these three elements:

1. An unlawful application of force
2. Against the person of another
3. Resulting in either bodily injury or an offensive touching

Aggravated battery (or aggravated assault) is usually classified as a serious felony-grade offense. This type of charge is likely to be sought when a battery or assault causes serious bodily injury or permanent disfigurement. In some states, if you kick someone when you have shod feet (i.e., when you are wearing shoes), that may constitute an aggravated battery or aggravated assault—especially if that person is on the ground. Alternatively, other statutes recognize different levels of injury by classifying them in ascending order of seriousness: first degree (most serious), second or third degree (less serious).

"Reasonable Force" Parameters

You *must* use only force that appears reasonably necessary to prevent harm to yourself or another. You *must not* use force that is likely to cause death or serious bodily injury unless you reasonably believe you will be maimed or killed. Should you use more force than is necessary, you will lose the privilege of self-defense.

Once again, for nondeadly force, the law generally recognizes that a person may use such force as reasonably necessary to thwart the imminent use of force against that person, short of deadly force. Understand that you may also step into the shoes of a third party to intervene using and meeting a specific state's standard. The standard of reasonable force to which you are held will be that of a reasonably prudent person (found in the geographic area of the incident). What this means is the average juror may not—more likely *will not*—understand or fully appreciate the physical countermeasures you took. To absolve you of excessive force allegations, you must articulate why you used anatomical targeting to stop the threat.

An expert witness can bolster your argument by educating the jury about the nature of violent attacks and physical dangers. Remember that most untrained people, including your average jurors, conjure up images of violent action movies and police dramas when they think of counterviolence. You can only argue and present what you perceived to be a potential or actual threat. The court will infer from both circumstances and evidence what you did. You must highly influence this inference by your explanation of your actions (assuming your actions were justified) to prevent the aggressor from becoming the victim in the court's eyes and you the guilty perpetrator. Your actions must parallel and support your statements. Your statements must do the same for your actions.

Legal Questions You Could Face

Legally, self-defense is an affirmative defense. This means you admit to (counter) attacking the aggressor. You have the burden of proving you acted in self-defense and, crucially, that *you were not the aggressor*. To explain your actions, you need only to have a reasonable belief regarding the violent nature and danger of the other person's actions. Importantly, apparent necessity—not actual necessity—will suffice for a sustainable self-defense explanation.

You will have to articulate why you had no choice but to use counterviolence. You will need to explain the following four reasonable beliefs for a self-defense claim:

1. Intent: The suspect had the stated or evident goal of harming you.
2. Capability: The suspect had the prowess or tools to harm you.
3. Opportunity: The suspect had the proximity to harm you.
4. Lack of preclusion: You did not have the option to retreat.

The legal justification for your self-defense actions may center on (1) how well you can articulate the reasons for your actions and (2) whether your counterviolence was warranted under the standard of reasonableness.

To justify your actions, you'll likely have to explain the following in a police statement and, possibly, on a witness stand:

- Your ability to recognize the difference between normal movements and attack movements.
- Your preexisting learned knowledge of threats. In other words, you'll likely need to explain your observations when another person 1) presents countermeasures against your initial nonviolent safety measures, 2) develops the proximity and ability to attack, and 3) duplicates well-known threatening attack-movement patterns.
- Your reasonable belief that, given the totality of the circumstances, you faced imminent and immediate physical danger.
- Your use of preemptive self-defense to stop the aggressor just before he could launch his attack. If you use preemptive counterviolence, you must describe why an attack was not just possible, but it was probable (i.e., when the aggressor acts in a manner consistent with attack movements).
- Your reasons why preclusion (retreat) was not available.
- That you acted with objectively reasonable counterforce. Remember that fear and adrenaline can affect your actions when confronting danger. This may explain any inconsistencies between your perceptions and statements when compared with video of the actual incident.
- Your goal and intent of stopping the threat. You had no wish to cause wanton injury.
- That you recognized the probable outcome of not stopping the threat. As examples you can articulate, these may include the following: suffering a fractured eye orbit or broken nose, having your head smashed on the ground, or being stomped. For this point, you may have to provide answers to the following use-of-force questions:
  1. Was it necessary to kick and severely damage the other party's knee?
  2. Why did you attack the other party's eyeball?

3.   After you kneed the other party in the head, why did you stomp on his ankle?

4.   Why after disarming the other party and creating distance did you shoot him?

- That you did not create the violent confrontation.

Here are some interrelated questions you may face from the police and prosecutor:

- Couldn't you have precluded (left) the situation?
- Did you instigate the dispute?
- Why didn't you summon the police?
- How did you know or prove the other party was going to attack you?
- Why did you use that level of force?
- Didn't you intend to purposefully injure the other party?
- You train in krav maga to injure people, correct?

Using a retzev counterattack will invite acute legal scrutiny. For the average kravist, a retzev counterattack of continuous explosive counterviolence is usually completed in as few as two to three seconds. In a violent crisis situation, there is no time to analyze what specific counterattack might be optimum. You'll need to defend yourself by counterattacking whatever part of the attacker's vulnerable anatomy is opportune to stop him.

Should you decide to make a statement, it may be advisable that you provide preemptive answers to the possible police or prosecutor questions listed above before you are asked. It also may be advisable to exercise your rights as delineated in a Miranda warning not to make any statements until you consult with your attorney or are in the presence of an attorney. Note that you should reflect on your analysis of the situation and subsequent actions as best you can before answering questions or making a statement. If possible, wait until your adrenaline has subsided. In the legal repercussions of a violent confrontation, the person who first goes on the record with a more compelling story is likely to receive the benefit of the doubt.

Sample Use-of-Force Explanations

With the caveat that the following sample explanations are not to be construed as formal legal advice, you might provide these types of answers regarding questions as to the reasonableness of your use of force. Here are four hypothetical situations.

- Example 1, when defending a punch: "I kicked him in the knee to stop him from punching me in my head. Obviously, hitting someone in the head is dangerous. I didn't want him to do it to me, and by the same reasoning, I didn't want to hit him in the head to stop him—so, instinctively I kicked his knee to stop him. It is well known that people suffer concussions and secondary brain injuries from hitting their heads on the ground after being struck in the head. Had he been able to hit me in the head, he could continue to attack and injure me."

- Example 2, when defending a choke: "I struck him in his eyeball as a distraction to stop him from choking me, which could have killed me."

- Example 3, when defending a tackle takedown: "I instinctively kneed him in the head as he dropped his level to come at my knees. He continued his aggressive actions, so I then stomped on his ankle to stop him from further attack. His stance and takedown attempt suggested he was trained to take people down to injure them. It is well known that people such as boxers, mixed martial arts fighters, and other types of people skilled in hand-to-hand combat train to get hit in the head and continue an assault. If he had taken me down, he could have mounted me to beat me, break my arms, or choke me. I also could have been attacked by other people while I was on the ground."

- Example 4, when disarming and shooting a gunman with his own gun: "I was forced to shoot him because after I disarmed him and created distance from the threat, he would not obey my commands to get back. Clearly, he wanted to injure or kill me."

Personally, I would give a statement, but if it seems the investigation is turning against me, I would tell the officer or detective that while I will fully cooperate, I need the counsel of a lawyer before making any additional statements.

Scrutiny of Your Self-Defense Training

In the courtroom, a trained person is often held to a higher standard of reasonableness than the average person. Your training will no doubt be brought to light by the prosecution or plaintiff's attorney and similarly by your own attorney. The prosecutor or plaintiff's attorney will represent that you have, by virtue of your training, a better understanding of the use of force. Perhaps, in a jury's mind, you have through your training acquired a magic pressure point or a series of noninjurious joint locks you could have summoned to stop the attacker. It is precisely this better understanding of the use of force that you must be able to articulate. You must clarify both what you did and why you did it. You used your training to your advantage in the violent incident; now you must use that training in court to justify your actions.

This cannot be emphasized enough: when defending yourself, you are only entitled to use the amount of force that is commensurate or proportional to the threat. Recall that this book's goal is to optimize your combatives so, paradoxically, your legal defense of your actions is easier, not more difficult. In other words, for a police officer, district attorney, or jury perceiving your actions, one superior knee strike that stops an attacker will appear more reasonable than three ineffective knee strikes. *So again, do a combative right the first time.* Be sure to keep in mind that, tempting as it might be to severely hurt or kill your assailant, you must make a deliberate and conscious decision, a real-time reasonable assessment, when to cease your counterattack. If you use counterviolence, you must believe the stakes are real and the aggressor is playing for keeps.

In conclusion, not only does a practical, reality-based threat-analysis method enable you to avoid danger and violence, it also helps you develop a legal and liability shield against arrest and prosecution, should you need to use counterforce. If you must resort to violence to protect yourself, you must be able to explain to a jury why and how you chose your actions and that there were no reasonable alternatives. This is counterbalanced against the understanding that any serious physical confrontation has the potential to seriously injure or kill you. Even if you prevail in criminal court, you are likely to face civil proceedings. Financial penalties might include compensating the injured party for lost earnings, medical bills, pain, and suffering, along with the prospective of a jury awarding punitive damages to teach you a lesson. Keep in mind that the burden of proof to demonstrate civil liability is less restrictive than a prosecutor's burden of proof. In a civil proceeding, it is necessary only to show that it is more likely than not that your actions caused physical injuries, mental anguish, and other losses.

New Jersey Self-Defense Statute Example

One of the defenses to assault or battery is a claim of self-protection, or self-defense. I will use my home state, New Jersey, as an example of a more stringent self-defense statute. New Jersey statute 2C:3–4(a) "Use of Force in Self-Protection" provides the following:

> *The use of force upon or toward another person is justifiable when the actor reasonably believes that such force is immediately necessary for the purpose of protecting himself against the unlawful force by such other person on the present occasion.*[1]

When claiming self-defense, it is critical to show that you acted with objectively reasonable force, as will be discussed in more detail. Section 2C:3–4 does not provide a defense for all forms of self-protection. While the law allows for some flexibility, in New Jersey, if you respond with deadly force when faced with what appears to be a minor confrontation, the provisions of section 2C:3–4 would likely not apply.

---

[1] https://law.justia.com/codes/new-jersey/2013/title-2c/section-2c-3-4/

In addition to requirements of objectively reasonable force, New Jersey's self-defense law also includes other important limitations. A self-defense claim is *inapplicable* in the following situations[2]:

- The use of counterforce against an owner or occupant of a property where the owner or occupant is lawfully using force in self-defense or defense of property to eject you.
- A situation where you provoked the original attack.
- In the case of deadly force, a situation in which you could have avoided the use of force with "complete safety" by retreating. In New Jersey, you are not required to retreat from your own dwelling prior to acting in self-defense, although limitations apply here as well.

An assault is purposeful if the person intended the injury to occur. A person causes an injury knowingly when that person is aware his or her actions will almost certainly cause bodily injury. New Jersey has enacted several assault categories. Simple assault is the most common charge in New Jersey. Simple assault charges arise when an individual attempts to do the following[3]:

1. Cause, or knowingly or recklessly cause, bodily injury to another,
2. Negligently cause bodily injury to another with a deadly weapon, or
3. Place someone in fear of imminent injury by menacing.

A simple assault is classified as a disorderly persons offense. If the simple assault stems from a mutual fight, then it's categorized as a petty disorderly persons offense. However, if an assault is more serious, such as an assault on a police officer, firefighter, or other protected class, or if the assault is conducted with a vehicle, it is classified as aggravated assault.

---

[2] https://law.justia.com/codes/new-jersey/2013/title-2c/section-2c-3-4/
[3] https://law.justia.com/codes/new-jersey/2013/title-2c/section-2c-12-1/

New Jersey Assault Summary Table[4]

Statutes	New Jersey Statutes 2C:12-1 (Assault)
	New Jersey Statutes 2C:33-2 (Disorderly Persons Offense)
Simple Assault	• An attempt to cause or knowingly or recklessly causes bodily injury to another person; or
	• A negligent act that causes bodily injury to another person with a deadly weapon; or
	• An attempt by physical menace to put another person in fear of imminent serious bodily injury.
	• Simple assault is a disorderly persons offense, a misdemeanor, punishable by up to six months in jail and/or a maximum $1,000 fine.
	• If the simple assault is committed in a fight with mutual consent, it is a petty disorderly persons offense, a misdemeanor, punishable by up to thirty days in jail.
Aggravated Assault	• A reckless act with a deadly weapon, causing bodily injury to another person.
	• An attempt to cause or an act that purposely causes bodily injury to another person with a deadly weapon.
	• An attempt to cause serious bodily injury to another person or cause such injury purposefully, knowingly, or under a negligent or reckless situation; or
	• Recklessly pointing a firearm at another person, whether or not the actor believes it to be loaded.
	• An individual charged with aggravated assault may face up to ten years in prison and a fine of up to $150,000.
Possible Defenses	• Self-defense.
	• Consent.

The penal consequences for assault and battery differ from state to state. Misdemeanor assault and battery charges may result in fines, community service, probation, or imprisonment for up to one year or possibly more. Repeat offenders are usually sentenced more severely. Felony assault convictions result in prison terms of five to twenty-five years.

Anatomical Targeting

A key tenet of krav maga is to attack whatever anatomical targets the aggressor presents. His punch attempt may leave a knee open to a side kick. His attempted rear

---

[4] https://statelaws.findlaw.com/new-jersey-law/new-jersey-assault-and-battery-laws.html

choke hold against you on the ground may leave his groin vulnerable. The kravist learns to laser in on these anatomical targets of opportunity. Within the range of possible targets are anatomical points that yield especially effective results—maximum effect.

The Israeli Krav Maga Advantage: Anatomical Targeting

- Utilize a well-timed, decisive preemptive attack, creating anatomical damage followed by additional combatives.

- Begin with the intent to injure and neutralize your opponent. Your goal is to achieve traumatic injury in the shortest time, using the most opportune route. A trained paroxysm of counterviolence is more likely to favorably conclude the situation.

- Target an assailant's vital soft tissue, chiefly the groin, neck, and eyes. Secondary targets include the kidneys, solar plexus, knees, liver, joints, fingers, nerve centers, and other smaller, fragile bones. In short, your rapid infliction of successive damage, mutilation, and wounds epitomizes the optimum use of counterviolence.

- Target the adversary's vulnerable anatomy, damage that anatomy, continue to damage it, and capitalize on debilitating him to move on to the next anatomical target as necessary.

- Use the closest weapon to attack the closest target. For example, don't kick with an inopportune leg if the other leg is closer to the opponent and your weight distribution and momentum allow you to use it.

- Inflict injury, which affords the opportunity to impose more injury. Recognize that an assailant might also attack these same targets on you and, accordingly, take measures to protect your own vital anatomy. A protective posture or stance is integral to krav maga training.

- Remember that the one who first imposes a debilitating injury and then follows through with additional combatives is usually the one who prevails.

Spinal reflexes govern the body's physical reaction to damage. While the human body is physically resilient, structural injury affects it in a somewhat predictable manner. Therefore, a kravist can generally predict how his counterattacks will affect the assailant's subsequent movements or capabilities. Strategically, inflicting a first-salvo injury against an adversary opens the door to unleash subsequent injurious counterattacks. For example, when an attacker is hit in the face, usually his head will jolt backward. This exposes his throat and neck to attack while also forcing his pelvis forward, exposing his groin and thus providing a target for further attack. As emphasized, the optimum way to end a violent conflict is to injure the opponent rapidly and repeatedly as necessary.

Krav maga, at its core, does not so much reflect "fighting" prowess (exchanging blows and absorbing physical punishment) as instead the ability to physically damage the adversary. In a fight, experienced combatants understand that specific defensive tactics rarely work or are applied. Rather, it is your offensive capabilities that are paramount. Does this mean that you do not actually defend? No, because at the heart of effective krav maga lies the axiom that a defensive move instantly turns into an offensive move. For example, suppose an attacker throws a hook punch at you. Your blocking *defense* to the inside of his arm—done with maximum velocity and force—is really an *offensive* attack, a strike followed by continuing offensive techniques.

While the kravist should ideally possess a sizeable repertoire of offensive moves, some counterattacks have demonstrated themselves to be more useful than others. If I were asked to give a short list of the techniques I believe would prove most effective in the shortest amount of time, I would suggest the ones in the following ordered list. To put this in terms of approaches to a situation, I would always look for opportunities, for example, to use a straight or side kick against an opponent at the appropriate distance or to use an eye rake up close. In your training, condition yourself to think of drawing these dirty dozen krav arrows from your quiver first.

Krav Maga's Dirty Dozen of Combatives

1) Linear kicks and knees: Straight kicks and knees, low-line side kicks, rear defensive kicks

2) Low roundhouse kicks

3) Linear straight punches and palm-heel strikes

4) Hook palm-heel strikes and inside chops

5) Eye rakes and gouges

6) Groin strikes

7) Horizontal #1 elbow

8) Over-the-top #8 elbow

9) Rear elbow strike #3, outside chops, forearm strikes

10) Chokes

11) Bites

12) Takedowns (Let gravity do its work without the defender going to the ground.)

Developing Power and Balance for Maximum Effect

This section continues to emphasize the *how* of effective krav maga, this time in terms of how you use your body for the best outcomes.

Israeli krav maga is designed to work for anyone regardless of athleticism, skill, size, or gender. As noted, there are a few elementary techniques you can perform instinctively and apply to a wide variety of situations. Importantly, you need not master more than a few combatives to become a kravist or competent krav maga fighter capable of defeating any type of unarmed or armed attack or threat.

While there are no set solutions for ending a violent confrontation, there are preferred methods using retzev. Krav maga uses retzev to prevail by overwhelming an assailant to complete the defense. It cannot be emphasized enough that, to adopt and streamline the krav maga method, you personalize the techniques to make them your own. For example, you may like a straight lead kick followed by a straight (same-side) lead punch. Or you may prefer a rear straight kick followed by a rear straight punch. You may prefer two alternating horizontal elbow #1 strikes or, instead, a lead horizontal elbow strike #1 followed by a rear over-the-top elbow strike #8 combination. (These elbow strikes are all spelled out in this book. See the section named "Combative Family #4: Elbow Strikes.") Choose the ballistic strikes and other combatives you feel most comfortable with and that give you the greatest confidence.

Self-defense involves different phases that are best categorized by the distance or proximity opponents maintain as the attack evolves. From a long or medium range, opponents have unhindered movement to batter one another, usually involving long kicks, medium punches, and other hand strikes. From a short range, knees, elbows, head butts, and biting become options. This includes a variety of standing entanglements involving medium and short strikes, trapping, clinching, throws, takedowns, and standing joint locks, all combined for "close retzev." A final phase may occur when both opponents lock up to unbalance one another to the ground, involving medium and short combatives combined with locks and chokes.

As noted, movement on the ground is different from standing movement. The nature of ground survival can allow one opponent superior control and positioning; the other opponent cannot run or evade as he might while standing. Krav maga ground survival is best defined as "what we do up, we do down," with additional specific ground-fighting capabilities. We employ many of our standing combatives on the ground, including groin, eye, and throat strikes in combination with joint breaks and dislocations designed to maim the adversary. So remember that what you learn to do standing is simply and effectively modified for ground survival applications.

The best way to practice these combatives—as with all techniques—is in stages. Each stage must be isolated, practiced, and perfected. As you master each stage, you can then combine them for the whole combative. A full-length mirror can help you monitor your form.

Many parts of your body, including your hands, forearms, elbows, knees, shins, and head can be used as personal weapons. There is a distinct advantage in using the hard parts of your body such as your elbows, knees, and feet as weapons against your attacker's vulnerable body parts. Optimized striking involves keeping the body's muscles relaxed until just before your limb impacts the opponent. By making the body rigid, using a strong, balanced base a fraction of a second before impact, you generate maximum speed to then instantly incorporate your body mass behind the strike.

As stressed, attacking an opponent's soft vital tissue, especially the eyes, throat, and groin, is one of the surest ways to end the fight, and krav maga emphasizes these targets. You know your body's sensitive spots. If you inadvertently poke yourself in the eye without closing your eyelid, you will immediately feel your eyeball tense and begin to water. If you have inadvertently hit yourself in the groin or landed on a bicycle bar the wrong way, you know the result. Lightly tap yourself in the throat and you will feel the sensitivity immediately.

Remember that striking someone in the throat can have serious and perhaps fatal consequences. Of course, this is why we are so adamant in protecting our own throats, along with our other vital body parts. These specific strikes must only be used if you are in fear for your life and limb. These strikes are commonly employed from an intermediate range, which is punching range. As with other upper-body strikes, hip and weight movement are essential to delivering reach and power to take advantage of your body's core strength and mass behind the combatives. The striking hand or forearm must also be properly positioned and aligned.

Proper krav maga techniques do not rely on strength. The power behind combatives derives from correct execution, not from body size or muscular strength. Many people think of hand-to-hand combat as exactly that: using your fists to strike at an opponent. Yet krav maga teaches you to use every part of your body—from the head to the foot—as a tool to deliver strikes. Regardless of your body size or muscular strength, you can deliver powerful strikes with your hands and elbows. Precise execution of a punch or elbow strike will generate much more impact than muscling your way through.

For a great overview and incisive explanation of the physics underlying krav maga and martial arts applications, I highly recommend *Fight Like a Physicist* (YMAA, 2015), by Jason Thalken, PhD. Physics dictates that acceleration times mass equals force. Your strike will generate more force if you accelerate as you extend your arm to put all your body weight (mass) behind an upper-body strike. The same is true, of course, for executing a lower-body combative. Alternatively stated, any combative strike will have more force if you accelerate your speed in combination with a total body-weight shift as you extend your personal weapons through your target.

The difference between high-momentum strikes and high-energy strikes is that high-momentum strikes drive an opponent backward. Momentum is your weight combined with how fast your limb strikes. Kinetic energy is the measure of tissue damage you inflict on an impact area. Israeli krav maga emphasizes transferring both momentum and kinetic energy through a strong, small, robust striking point, as illustrated in the following photos.

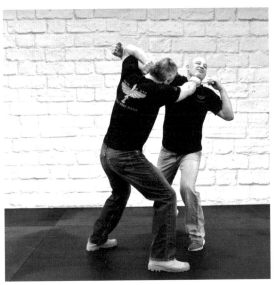

Straight punch using the first two knuckles (pointer and middle fingers) in counterattacking against a hook punch.

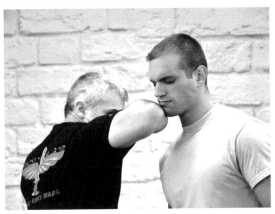

Horizontal elbow strike using the top of the ulna bone (just below one's elbow tip).

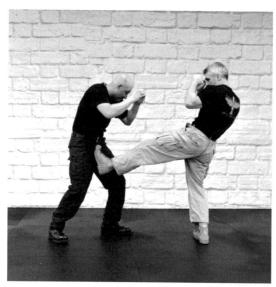 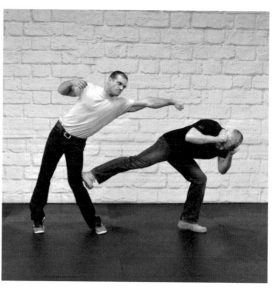

Straight kick delivered with the ball of a curled foot.   Low side kick delivered with the heel.

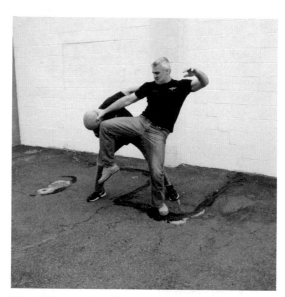

Straight knee using the patella (kneecap).

To increase the damage of a strike, create maximum velocity as well as follow-through. Follow-through involves farther extension of the striking limb, enabled by pivoting correctly. You can see this in the following photo series. Note the pivot of the base leg, or nonkicking leg.

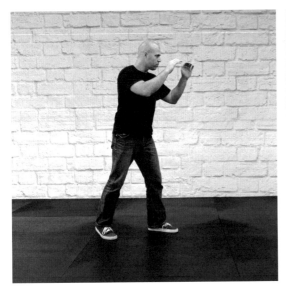 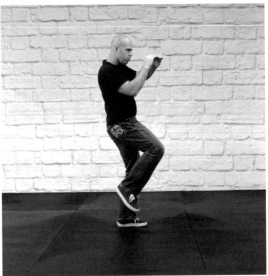

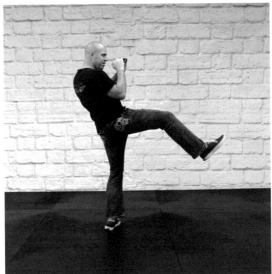

For the straight kick (or knee), pivot on the ball of the foot of the base leg for maximum power and reach. This harnesses the full power of your hips and body weight.

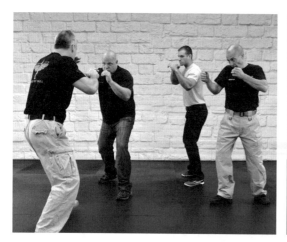 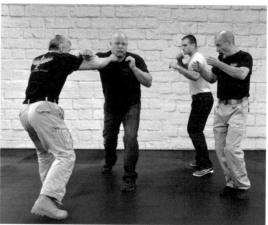

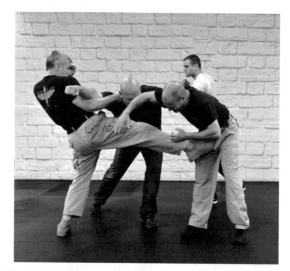

For the straight kick (or knee), pivot on the ball of the foot of the base-leg for maximum power and reach. This harnesses the full power of your hips and body weight.

What would you rather deliver: one superior debilitating kick or multiple inferior, ineffective kicks that do not incapacitate an attacker immediately? Certainly this question becomes more prominent if multiple attackers are introduced. More often than not, Imi Lichtenfeld faced multiple assailants. Every combative had to count. There might not be time or space to deliver a secondary combative because another attacker might set upon the defender immediately. This is not to say that multiple combatives might not be warranted against an attacker; it's simply that you might not have the chance to deliver another one.

Along with efficacy, with the proliferation of cameras, both stationary and through handheld devices, you may well be filmed defending yourself. What will appear more reasonable in a case of self-defense to a prosecutor or jury? One well-placed kick or three ineffective kicks? From an objectively reasonable force standard, obviously, one kick is the answer. Remember: juries often do not understand the reality of self-defense—that it often takes more than one combative to defeat a determined attacker—and jurors might expect one combative counterattack to suffice. Any more than one or two combatives and you might be considered to have employed excessive force.

Extreme force driven through vulnerable anatomy creates injury. Combative strikes harvest the largest possible load of kinetic energy to then drive it through the opponent's targeted anatomy. This is achieved by harnessing the entire weight of the body to propel it, using a balanced movement through the target via a combative strike. The combative strike can only be optimized when you create sound structure, as the krav maga combatives depicted in this book demonstrate.

Good training partners will help you refine your combatives by sometimes working against you hard, as though your combatives had no effect, and other times with controlled training that simulates how the body would react when affected by traumatic injuries. Economy of both combative motion and targeting seeks to create damage every time you make contact with the opponent.

CHAPTER 3

Upper-Body Combatives

Combatives Family #1: Straight Punches, Palm Heels, and Web Strikes

The descriptions in the following combatives sections include a few examples of the actual technique and its correct execution. Many will include a description of the results if the execution is not done correctly. In studying all of the following combatives, the reader should have our equation firmly in mind:

$$Correct\ Technique + Correct\ Execution = Maximum\ Effect$$

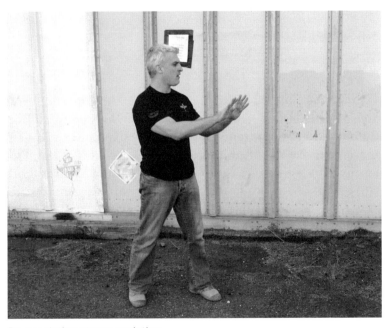

De-escalation stance variation.

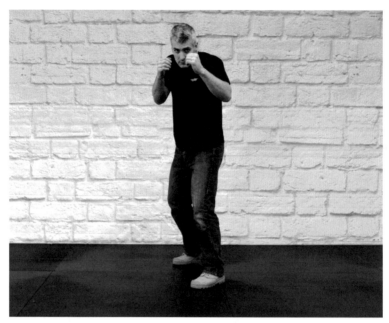

Left outlet stance.

Proper technique starts with a strong stance. In Israeli krav maga, you learn two basic stances:

1. The left outlet stance
2. The right outlet stance

Both stances use the same leg and arm positioning. The difference between them is that in one your body is bladed right, and in the other your body is bladed left. Your outlet stance protects your groin from incoming strikes and gives you a strong base of support to launch defensive and offensive strikes with your arms or legs. From this position you can easily launch your own kick with either your lead or rear leg. You must be fluid in changing from one stance to the opposite, as this will be a key in successfully applying retzev. Many common mistakes include positioning the hands improperly, placing the feet too close or too far apart, remaining flatfooted, blading improperly, hunching down, and failing to tuck the chin.

Since the majority of people are right-handed, we usually teach the left outlet stance first, placing the strong side to the rear. However, because Israeli krav maga relies on retzev, you must be fluid and comfortable using both the left and right outlet stances. For the left outlet stance, blade your body by turning your feet approximately 30 degrees to your right, with your left arm and left leg forward. (From a neutral or casual stance, you can also turn 30 degrees to your left to come into a right regular outlet stance, so your right leg and arm are forward.) You are resting on the balls of both your feet with your rear foot in a comfortable and balanced position. Your feet should be roughly parallel, with about 55 percent of your weight distributed on the ball of your front foot and the remaining 45 percent of your weight distributed on the ball of your rear foot.

Your arms are positioned in front of your face (but not blocking your eyes) and bent slightly forward at approximately a 60-degree angle between your forearms and your upper arms. To place your arms properly, assume the correct footwork for the stance and keep your elbows at your sides. Once your feet are properly positioned to blade your torso and establish a balanced, comfortable base that allows you to remain on the balls of your feet, simply raise your hands up to your eyebrows. This positions the hands to defend the head and execute counterattacks. You will note that in some of the photo series, the defender's hands are shoulder level initially but immediately raise up to eyebrow level as the distance to the opponent closes. From this stance you will move forward, laterally, and backward, moving your feet in concert. The key to instinctively reacting as quickly as possible is remaining on the balls of both feet while *not thinking about reacting, only impulsively countering the attack.*

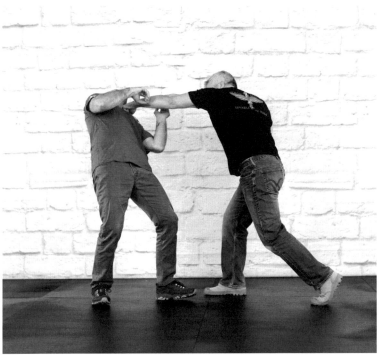

Rear (cross) straight punch: note the full pivot with the ball of the rear foot. This is for maximum reach and power transfer. The chin is tucked and the cover hand is up.

The bones in your hand are small and fragile. If you don't use proper alignment, you can easily break them when striking against hard bone. To make a fist, curl your fingers into your palms, placing your thumbs on top of your index fingers, not inside of your fist. Keep the back of your hand in line with your wrist and forearm. Any bend other than a slight downward angle of the wrist can cause serious damage, especially a rotation to the left or right, which takes the wrist out of its natural alignment. Hitting a target with your wrist misaligned can break the bones in your wrist and your hands. Whenever possible, aim for soft-tissue targets, lock your wrist, and make contact using the first two knuckles. To strengthen your wrists and knuckles for punching, do push-ups on your knuckles. The form is depicted in the following photo.

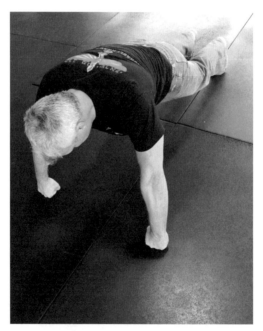

Knuckles and wrist aligned for a straight punch using either arm.

Regardless of the type of punch you deliver, shift your body weight forward to deliver the strike. Your forward weight displacement allows you to place all your body mass behind the punch, thereby connecting with greater force. When you practice punching, do not lock your elbows. Elbow hyperextension injuries are often caused by punching forcefully in the air or without resistance. When not making contact with a training pad (or sparring partner), extend your arms about 90 percent as you deliver a strike. Strong pad and bag work will accustom your striking limbs to impact, while building strength and stamina. Heavy bags are particularly useful for this type of training. Here are some pointers for striking effectively:

- **Use your entire body**. As you strike, move the entire body in concert. Rather than striking with only your hand or elbow, use your entire torso. As you propel all your strength and body weight through the strike, you'll maximize its impact.

- **Breathe**. Exhale as you deliver the strike. Some people like to use a blood-curdling cry as they strike. Either technique—the cry or exhale—will prepare your body for both delivering a strike and receiving a strike. Exhaling facilitates oxygen transfer to your muscles, tempers your movements to keep you in control, and creates a vacuum to defend against a counterstrike.

- **Aim for vulnerable anatomy**. You'll get more bang for your effort if you strike at vulnerable anatomy. Aiming for the body's soft tissues—the neck, groin, and other sensitive areas—helps increase the effectiveness of your strike.

Straight Punch

Lead Straight Punch

The lead straight punch is fast and direct. Aim for the nose, jaw, or throat. Stand in the left outlet stance with your hands in loose fists. Step forward with your left foot while quickly drawing your rear heel slightly in and back. Do not jump at the same time with both feet. There is a pause of a fraction of a second between the steps as your entire body mass launches forward. Simultaneously extend your left arm, jabbing your fist toward your target. Do not wind up; initiate with your arm out directly from the shoulder. Remember that the hand always leads to the body to prevent telegraphing. As your arm extends to deliver the punch, tighten your fist. Make contact with your hand parallel to the ground. If you deliver a palm-heel strike, your hand should be perpendicular to the ground. Wrist alignment is crucial to avoid injury.

Remember that you can perform knuckle push-ups to strengthen your upper body and wrists. When you strike an opponent with your fist, the soft tissue and bones in your hand compress to absorb some energy from the impact. If your hand and wrist are aligned properly to better absorb the impact, obviously you reduce the risk of injuring your hand. (Similarly, your foot compresses when delivering a straight kick, which is why we use the ball of the foot, not the toes.) For the straight lead punch or palm-heel strike, raise your left shoulder and tuck your chin to protect your jaw and neck. After striking, return immediately to your left outlet stance.

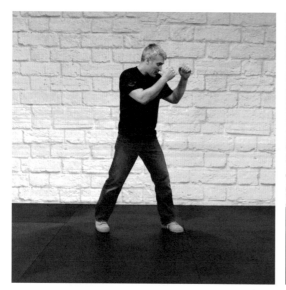 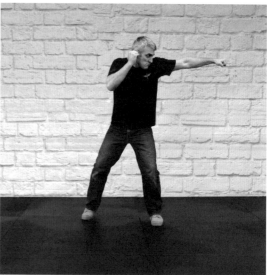

Lead straight punch.

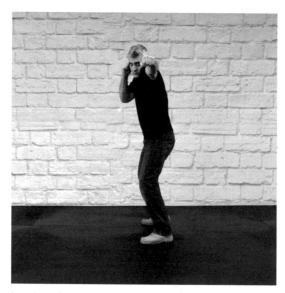

Lead straight punch (front view).

Rear Straight Punch

Similar to the lead punch, the rear straight punch technique best targets the nose, jaw, or throat. Stand in the left outlet stance with your hands in loose fists. Pivot your right leg slightly onto the ball of the foot as you drive your hips, rear shoulder, and arm forward toward your target. Tuck your chin into your right shoulder to protect it from an incoming strike. If you move both feet together while pivoting on the rear leg, your full body weight propels the punch forward for maximum power.

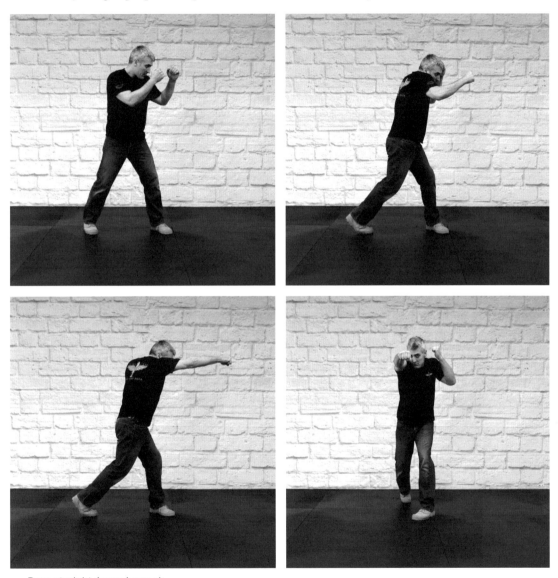

Rear straight (cross) punch.

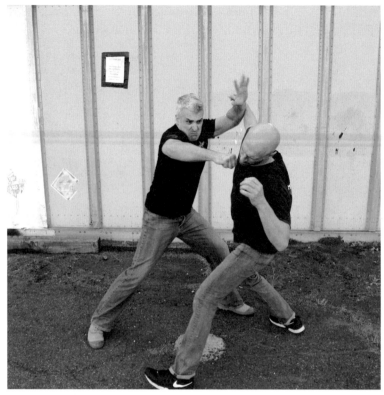

Rear straight (cross) punch (combined with opposite arm interception/deflection) used in defending a hook punch.

Straight Palm-Heel Strike

When using this direct and fast strike, aim for the nose, jaw, or throat. The strike is similar to the straight punch in terms of footwork, weight redistribution, and chin positioning. It is an effective intermediate-range strike, particularly for those who are not confident in the strength of their wrists and fists to execute regular punches. Remember: by curling up your wrist to expose the palm heel, you concede about three to four inches in strike reach when delivering a palm-heel strike as opposed to a straight punch with a closed fist.

Lead Straight Palm-Heel Strike

Starting from your regular outlet stance, make a palm heel by either tightly curling your fingers and pressing your thumb close to your hand or keeping your fingers open and bent back slightly to expose the palm heel. Your knuckles should be facing upward.

Pivot your right leg slightly onto the ball of the foot as you drive your hips, rear shoulder, and arm forward toward your target. Tuck your chin into your right shoulder to protect it from an incoming strike. Note: You can combine this technique with a subsequent eye rake.

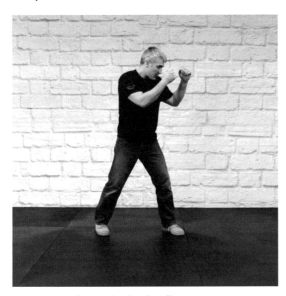 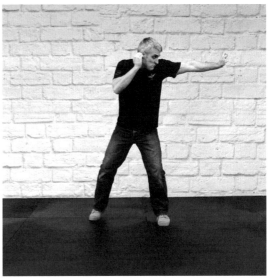

Lead straight palm-heel strike.

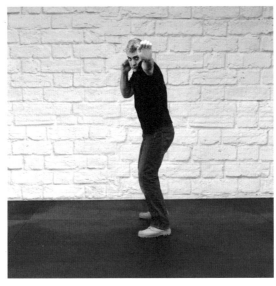

Lead straight palm-heel strike (front view).

Rear Palm-Heel Strike

Like the straight punch, this is also a direct and fast strike. As with the lead palm-heel strike, aim for the nose, jaw, or throat. Stand in the left outlet stance with your hands in loose fists. Pivot your right leg slightly onto the ball of the foot as you drive your hips, rear shoulder, and arm forward toward your target. Tuck your chin into your right shoulder to protect it from an incoming strike. Note: You can combine this technique with a subsequent eye rake.

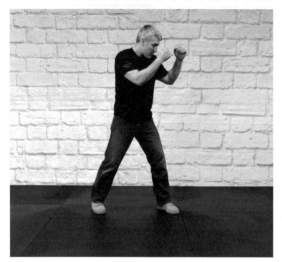 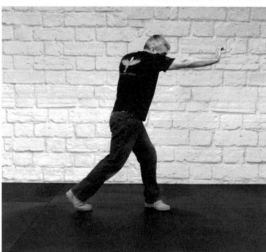

Rear straight (cross) palm-heel strike.

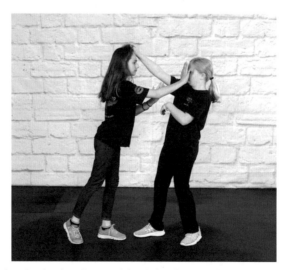

Rear straight (cross) palm-heel strike used in defending a hair grab. Note: The fingers of the striking hand are straight and not curled, an option if more comfortable for the striker. Compared to a straight punch, the palm-heel strike is less likely to injure the defender's hand. This makes it an effective option for young people who may need to defend against bullies or other aggressors.

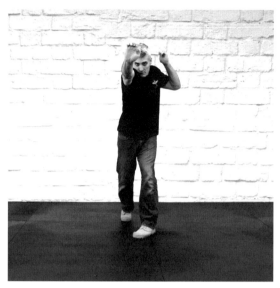

Rear straight (cross) palm-heel strike (front view).

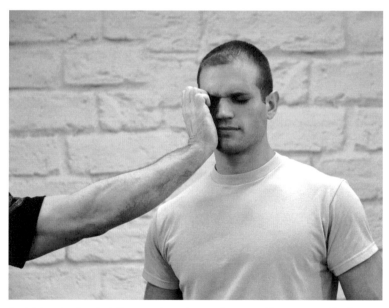

The rear straight palm-heel strike can target anywhere on the opponent's face—except the teeth, which can injure your hand.

The Beginnings of Your Personal Retzev

You can combine both the lead and rear punches or palm-heel strikes into a highly effective left-right combination. Begin with the lead punch, as it will reach the target more quickly than the rear punch. Withdraw the punching arm quickly into your fighting stance to maintain your defensive and offensive capability. As soon as you land the lead punch and begin to retract your lead arm, launch your rear punch. The momentum of drawing the lead punch back will help draw the rear punch forward, creating more impact. Think of punch combinations, especially the "one-two" straight punch combination, as alternating pistons in their coordinated movement.

If you must retreat, you can still stun your attacker with a retreating punch. As you shuffle backward, launch a lead punch to keep an oncoming attacker at bay. Retreat with the rear foot, followed by the lead foot, as the lead arm simultaneously extends to punch.

Short Inverted Punch

This quick punch using either arm allows you to cover a short distance to counterattack your opponent. Stand in a left outlet stance with your hands in loose fists. Punch as if you were connecting with a rear punch, except keep your pinkie side of the hand facing the ground. You may use this technique to defend against a straight punch by punching over the top of the incoming strike. The short inverted punch differs from the straight punch in that the knuckles are now vertical toward your target, and the elbow of the punching arm is close to the body. Against an outside hook punch, use the short inverted punch to move inside while executing a 360 outside block defense with your opposite arm. Your body explodes forward with a simultaneous defense and attack.

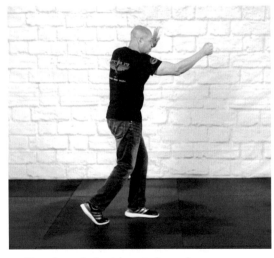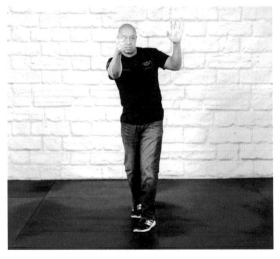

Rear (cross) short inverted punch.

As we have seen, push-ups are valuable in developing strength and alignment for the lead straight punch. Similarly, if you practice doing a one-handed plank, it will help you develop strength and form for the short inverted punch. The plank forces you to place your weight on your first two (striking) knuckles while properly aligning your wrist to support your weight.

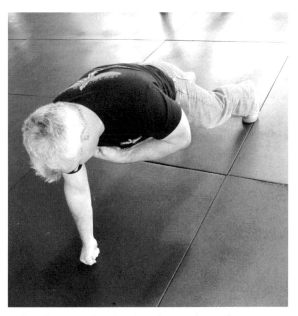

Wrist alignment for the short inverted punch.

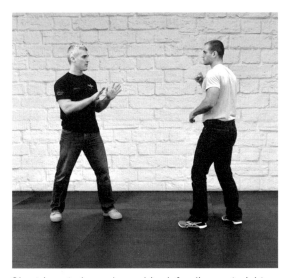

Short inverted punch used in defending a straight punch.

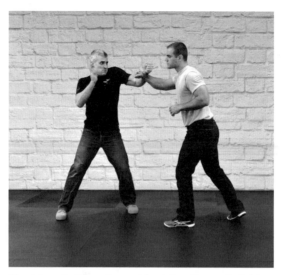

Short inverted punch used in defending a straight punch.

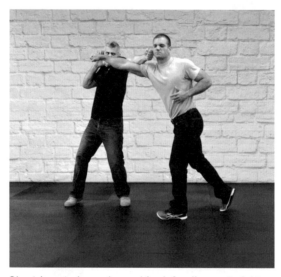

Short inverted punch used in defending a straight punch.

Half-Hook (Half-Roundhouse) Punch

Similar to the straight punches, this technique best targets the nose, jaw, or throat. Make contact with your first two knuckles while maintaining proper wrist alignment. The only difference is the angle of the punch, as you will keep your elbow slightly bent all the way through the punch to the point of making contact. The punch allows for you to counterattack from an off angle. Tuck your chin into your right shoulder to protect it from an incoming strike.

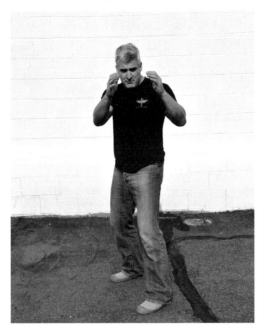
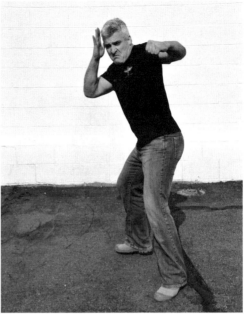

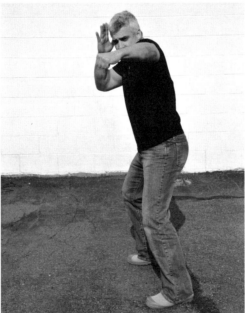

Lead half-hook punch.

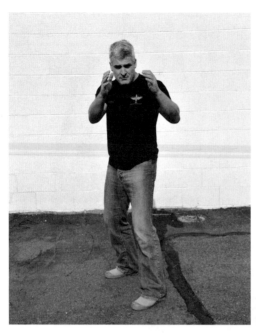 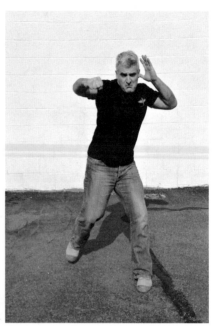

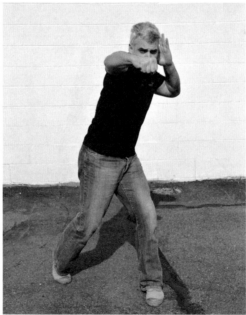

Rear half-hook punch.

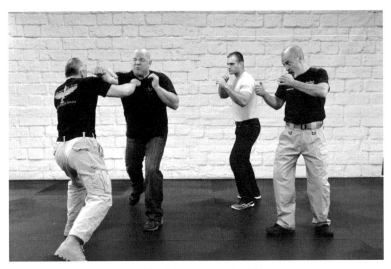

Rear half-hook punch used in defending a straight punch.

Over-the-Top Punch

The over-the-top punch attacks your opponent from a slightly vertical angle, slamming down on your opponent's eye socket, nose, or jaw. Your body movement is similar to that of the over-the-top elbow strike #8, where your striking arm moves high to low and slams down on your target. This strike is especially effective when you are able to trap an opponent's lead arm with your lead arm to bring down his defense, simultaneously delivering the strike to his exposed head.

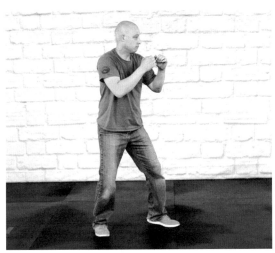
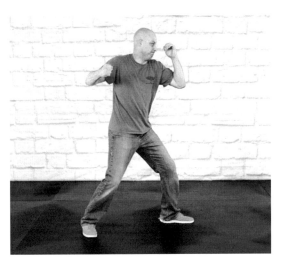

Over-the-top punch.

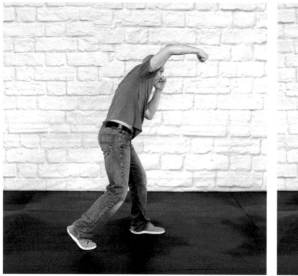
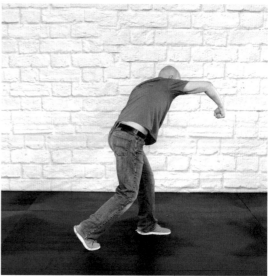

Over-the-top punch.

Knuckles Rake

The knuckles rake combative targets the eye ridge, temple, or nose. Contact is made with the middle three knuckles. The strike is made by raking down on the target. The photos represent the strike's motion, using a near-simultaneous attack and defense capacity against a rear double-handed choke with a push.

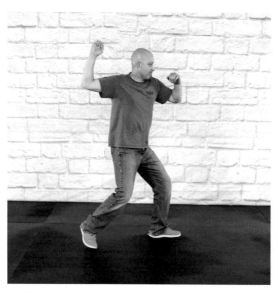
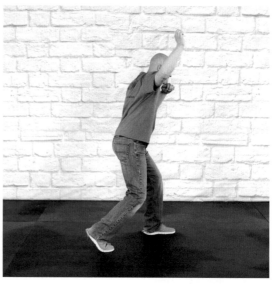

Knuckles rake.

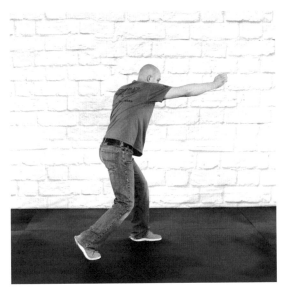 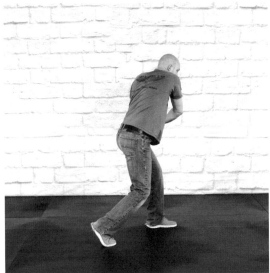

Knuckles rake.

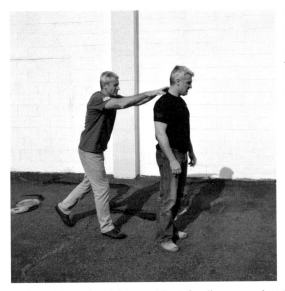 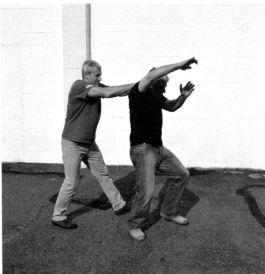

Knuckles-rake strike used in defending a rear hands choke.

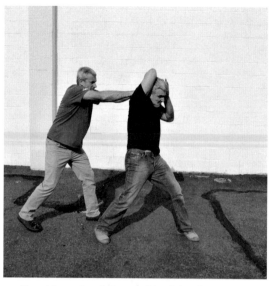
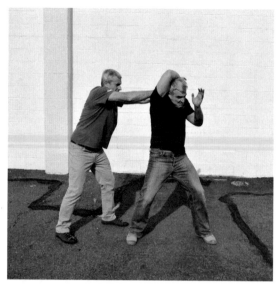

Knuckles-rake strike used in defending a rear hands choke.

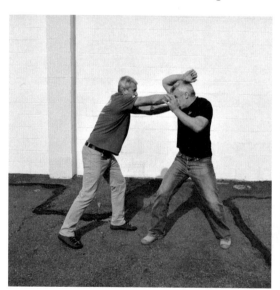
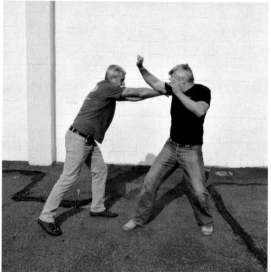

Knuckles-rake strike used in defending a rear hands choke.

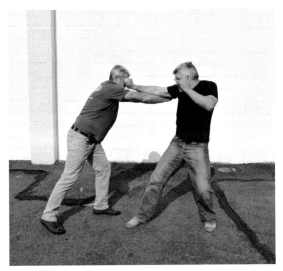 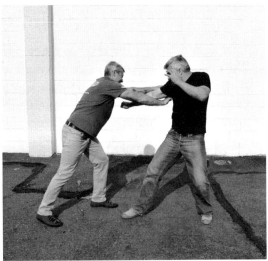

Knuckles-rake strike used in defending a rear hands choke.

Combative Family #2: Eye Claws, Rakes, Gouges, and Throat Strikes

Finger eye claws and rakes to the eyes can disable an opponent quickly and effectively. The eyeball can be collapsed with minimum pressure and easily scratched. Blinding or partially blinding an attacker sets up retzev follow-up strikes to end a confrontation quickly. One consideration, however, is avoiding this combative if you have cuts or abrasions on your fingers, as you could possibly contract pathogens from your opponent's eyes.

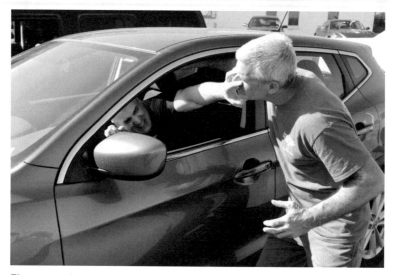

Finger eye claws and rakes used in defending a road-rage scenario.

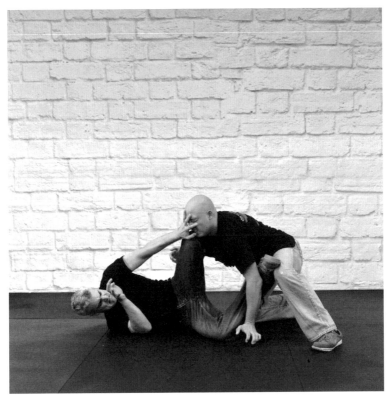

Lead straight eye gouge while on the ground.

For a multiple-finger strike, fold your fingers slightly inward toward your palm and spread them just enough so they do not touch. This will reduce the possibility of injuring them on impact. If the impact is hard, flexing the fingers inward will collapse them into their natural articulation. Note that the fingers are fragile and can easily be fractured, even when taking precautions. Execute the strike with a body movement similar to that of your straight punches, with the fingers making contact with the eyes. The second set of example photos shows a defender parrying a straight punch and immediately sliding his hand to deliver the multiple-finger strike to the attacker's eyes.

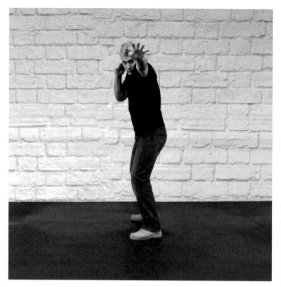
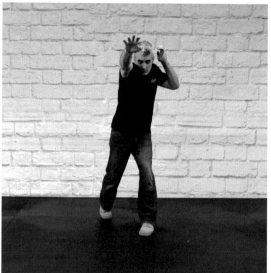

Lead straight eye rake.

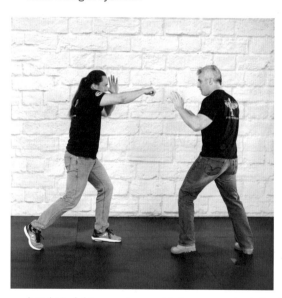
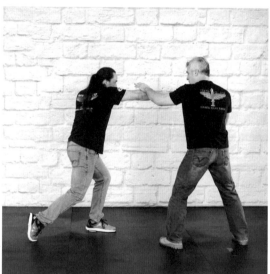

Lead straight eye rake used from a parry in defending a straight punch.

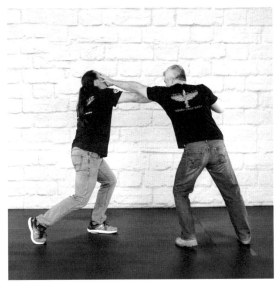

Lead straight eye rake used from a parry in defending a straight punch.

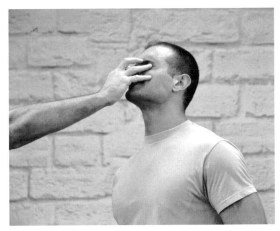

Lead straight eye rake. Close-up depicting digits slightly bent to prevent finger injuries.

Eye Gouge Using the Thumbs

You can also strike the eyes with your thumbs, penetrating the eye socket. This combative is certainly one of the most brutal and visceral in the krav maga arsenal. Use your opponent's cheekbone as a guide to strike with your palm heel, and then insert the thumb. Krav maga's rule of thumb (pardon the pun): if you can find the cheekbone, you can find the eye. This is particularly important if you are not in a position to see your attacker, such as in a ground-fighting situation or if it is dark. You can insert one or both of your thumbs into your opponent's eye sockets. In the hand-to-hand combat example depicted, one opponent traps the other's opponent's lead arm to facilitate a thumb gouge to the eye.

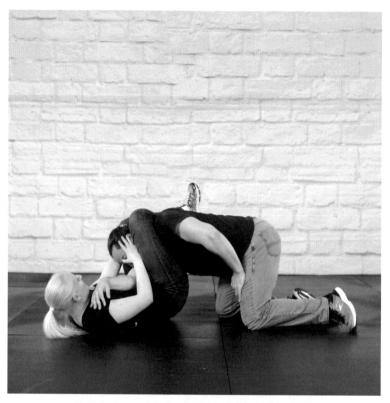

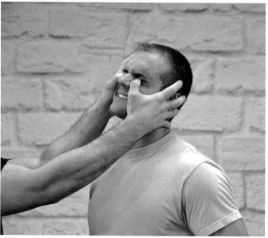

Two-thumb eye gouge using the cheek as a guide into the eye socket(s).

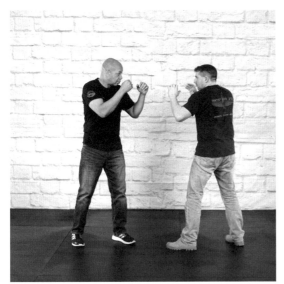
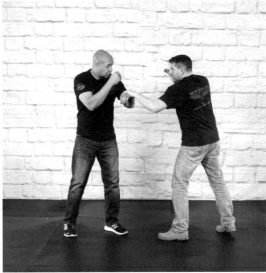
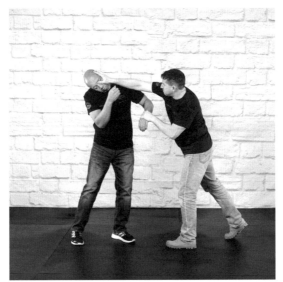

Arm trap and thumb eye gouge.

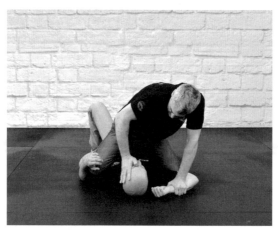

Arm trap and thumb eye gouge, ground version.

Web Strike to the Throat

When using this direct and fast strike, aim for the throat—specifically the windpipe. This strike must only be used when confronting an assailant who represents a deadly threat to you. If your timing and accuracy are correct, this can be a devastating first-strike option. The web strike uses the webbing of your hand between your forefinger and thumb to strike an opponent's throat and windpipe. Be sure to align your hand properly, as you could damage your thumb without proper targeting. By keeping the hand parallel to the ground, you create a thin striking tool capable of getting under an opponent's chin. Protect yourself by keeping your left hand up, and be prepared to launch another combative move.

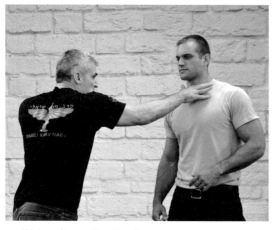
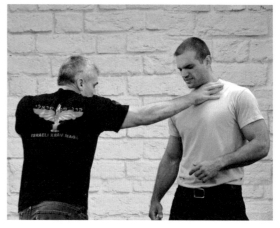

Web strike to the throat.

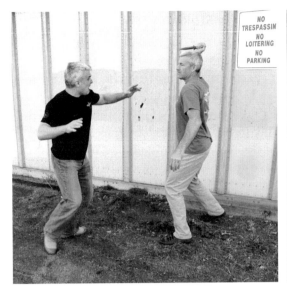
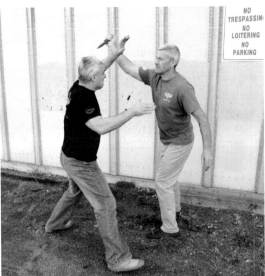
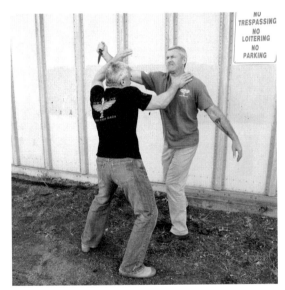

Web strike to the throat, used in defending against an overhead knife attack.

Combative Family #3: Groin Strikes

Hand and Elbow Groin Strikes

Hand and elbow groin strikes are highly effective follow-up strikes to the perpendicular rear elbow—or as independent strikes in their own right. Use this strike to target one of the body's most sensitive areas. One option to strike the groin is using a cupped hand. You may strike an opponent who is facing forward, to the side, or to the rear. By whipping your hand into the groin, you create a potent, debilitating blow. You can also use a hammer fist, punch, or vertical elbow strike #5 directly into the groin if your positioning allows it, as the various examples depict. Note that, if you defend immediately, groin strikes are highly effective against the popular mixed martial arts and jiu-jitsu mount and guard positions.

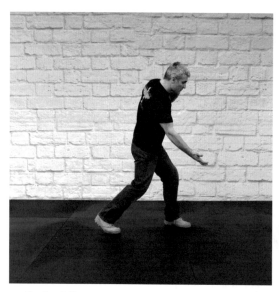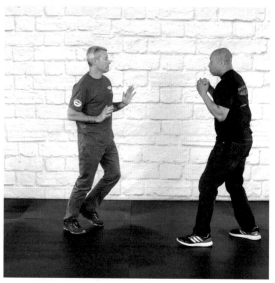

Groin strikes.

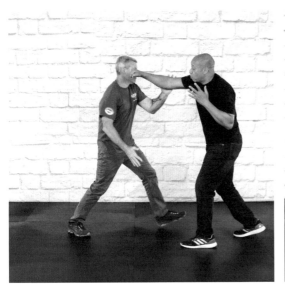 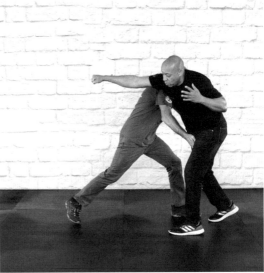

Groin strike used in defending a straight punch.

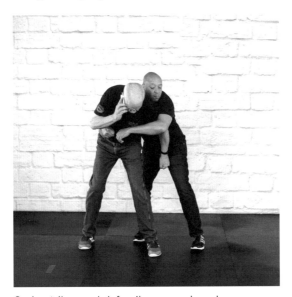

Groin strike used defending a rear bear hug.

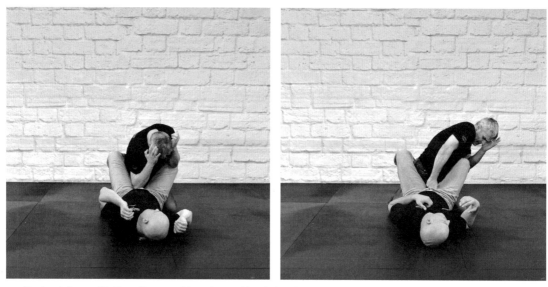

Groin strikes with the elbow and hand, used in defending the guard.

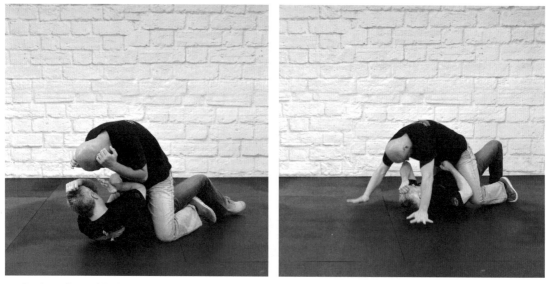

Groin strikes with the elbow and hand, used in defending the mount.

Combative Family #4: Elbow Strikes

Elbow Strikes

In this combative family you will learn krav maga's ten elbow strikes. The numbers of the strikes correspond with elbow techniques named throughout this book. As you deliver any elbow strike, you may either keep the hand of the striking arm open or clenched in a fist. If you keep the hand open, the muscles are less tense, allowing you to tighten them the split second before impact. A clenched fist tightens the forearm and active muscle groups to increase the strength of impact and help prevent injury—but it also makes the movement slightly slower because your energy is expended by tensing your muscles. Use the hand position that is most comfortable for you prior to delivering the elbow strike. You can achieve the best of both worlds by clenching the fist just prior to impact, while the elbow strike is in motion. This accelerates the strike and conserves energy because you do not tense your body longer than necessary.

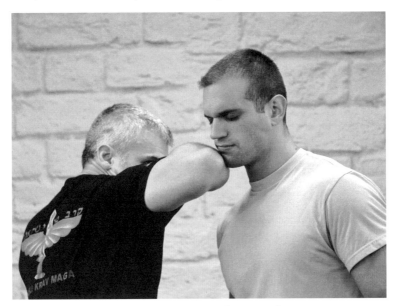

Horizontal right #1 elbow strike, close-up impact points.

Lead and Rear Horizontal Elbow Strikes

Horizontal elbows use the extremely hard surface just below the elbow tip to deliver a strong combative. The power and strength behind this strike is unparalleled. The elbow's path follows whatever opening or target your opponent gives you. Make impact with the target just below the tip of your elbow. Targets usually include the jaw, cheek, throat, and ear.

Lead Horizontal Elbow Strike #1

For a lead horizontal elbow strike, start in your left outlet stance with your hands protecting your face. Begin to pivot on the ball of your left foot in the direction of the strike, and lower your elbow parallel to the ground to initiate the combative movement. This is a simultaneous movement: you pivot your foot and move the arms from protecting your head to delivering the elbow combative. Connect with your target with your lead arm parallel to the ground and the hand pressed loosely against your upper chest. Make contact just below the tip of your striking elbow. As you deliver the lead horizontal elbow, pivot to the right on your lead foot in the same direction as the elbow combative so your lead heel nearly faces your target. As you pivot your heel, turn the rest of your body, but keep your eyes on the target.

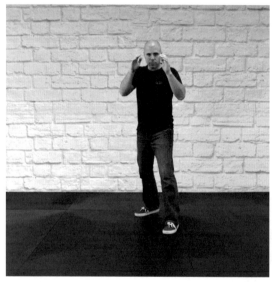 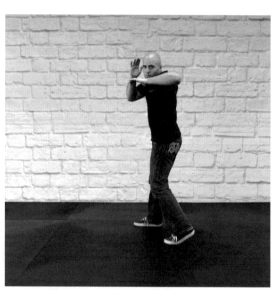

Lead horizontal elbow strike.

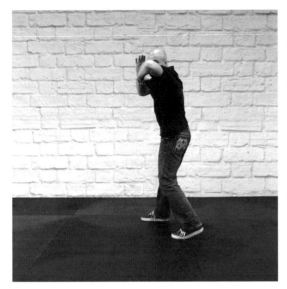 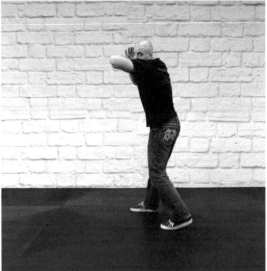

Lead horizontal elbow strike. Note full follow-through and pivot.

Rear Horizontal Elbow Strike #1

For a rear horizontal elbow strike, pivot to your left on the balls of your feet to deliver the rear strike as illustrated. This rear-arm horizontal elbow strike will have more power than your lead strike because your hip movement is greater, generating more power. Adjust your rear foot slightly to accommodate your lead foot's movement. Make contact just below the tip of your striking elbow. Keep your rear hand up in a fighting position.

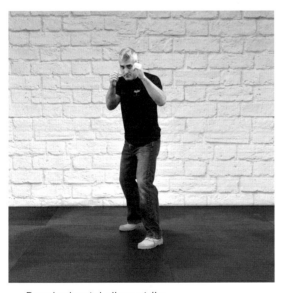 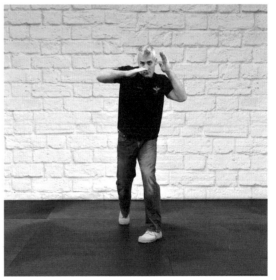

Rear horizontal elbow strike.

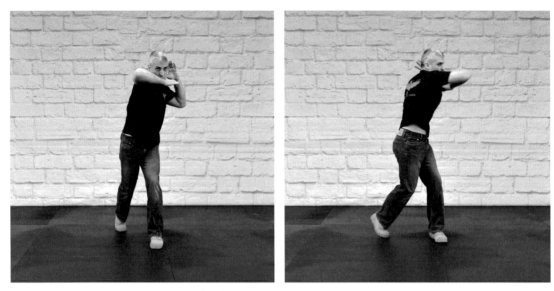

Rear horizontal elbow strike. Note full follow-through and pivot.

Lead and Rear Horizontal Elbow Strike Combination

These lead and rear horizontal elbow strikes are a natural, powerful combination. The lead horizontal elbow strike torques the body, forcing it to turn, thereby coiling it to deliver the rear horizontal elbow strike with extra power.

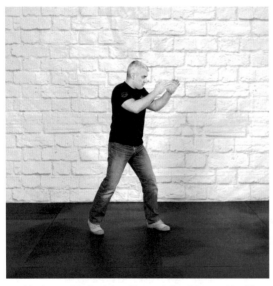
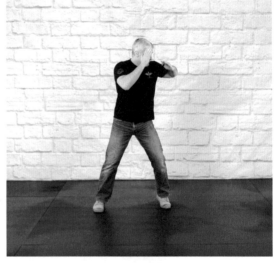

Horizontal left-right elbow strike #1 combination.

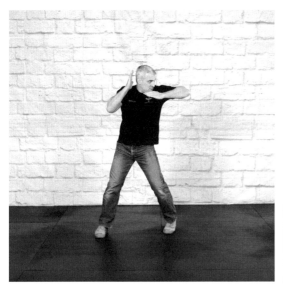 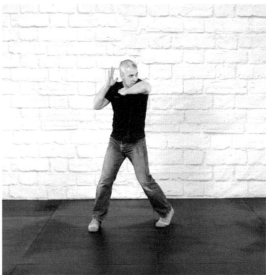

Horizontal left-right elbow strike #1 combination. Note full follow-through and pivot.

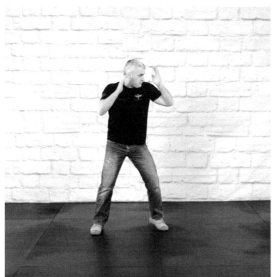 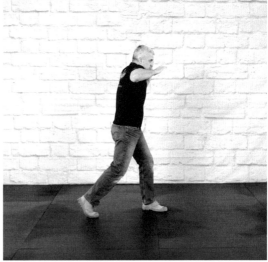

Horizontal left-right elbow strike #1 combination.

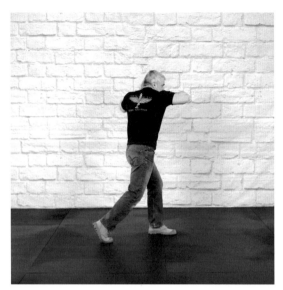 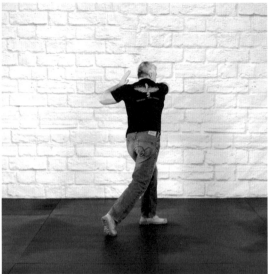

Horizontal left-right elbow strike #1 combination. Note full follow-through and pivot.

Lateral Elbow Strike #2 to the Side

A lateral elbow strike can attack an opponent who is standing to your side. Use this strike to target the face, jaw, and throat. Make contact with the tip of your striking elbow or just above the tip. In addition, depending on height and positioning, you can throw a modified horizontal elbow to the opponent's ribs, midsection, kidneys, and other targets of opportunity.

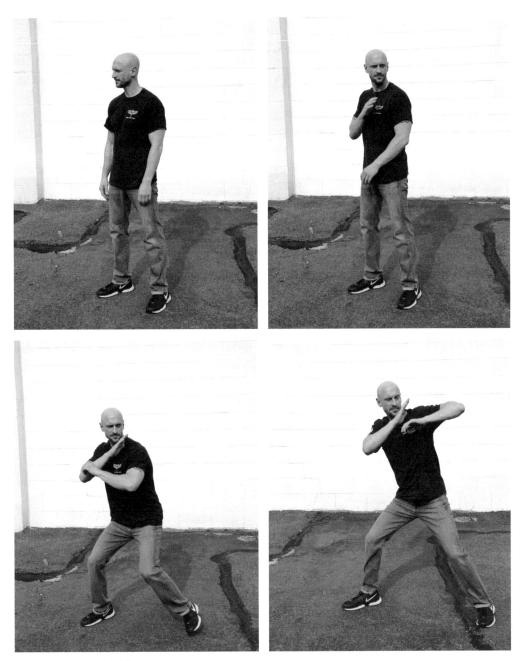

Lateral elbow strike #2.

Practice the technique from either your regular outlet stance or a passive stance. Your striking arm begins in a similar starting position as that of the horizontal elbow. Bring your striking arm parallel to the ground while making a fist, and draw your forearm close to your body. As with your other combative strikes, synchronize your lower- and upper-body movements. Bring the hand of your nonstriking elbow in front of your face on the same side as the striking arm. This covering movement further protects your face and sets you up for your next combative. As you deliver the strike, take a short side step forward in the same direction your elbow is traveling. This movement shifts the body weight behind the blow. For a right elbow strike, step to your right; for a left elbow strike, step to your left. As you step in the direction of your strike, extend the elbow as your triceps muscle makes contact. With your rear leg, take the same-size step as the lead leg, ending in roughly the same equidistant leg position from which you began.

Horizontal Elbow Strike #3 to the Rear

Begin in your regular outlet stance with your hands protecting your face. To execute the horizontal elbow strike #3 to the rear, turn your head to the rear, take a small step back to open up the hip, and deliver the strike to the opponent behind you. Targets usually include the jaw, cheek, throat, and ear. Your head must lead your body, while your hips generate power to deliver this short, compact strike. Bring your wrist into your body with your forearm parallel to the ground. For a right elbow, turn and step, opening with your right leg. This step will help you build momentum and power. Make contact with the tip of your striking elbow or just above the tip. As you deliver a horizontal elbow with your rear arm, pivot your core in the same direction as the elbow combative. This will increase the power of the strike. Keep your chin tucked.

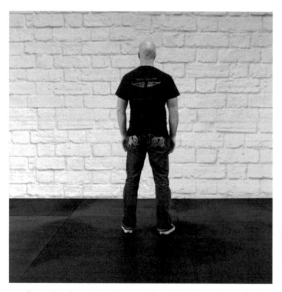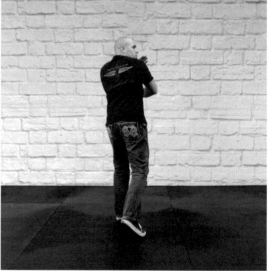

Rear horizontal elbow strike #3. Note that the head leads the body.

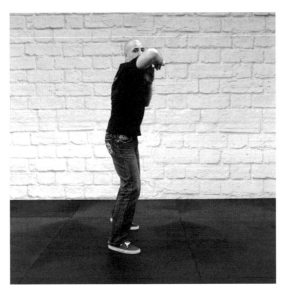

Rear horizontal elbow strike #3.

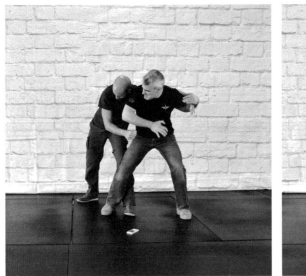 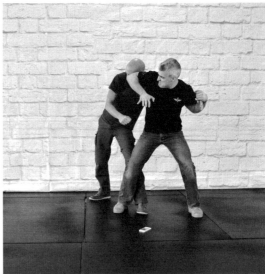

Rear horizontal elbow strike #3 used in defending an attempted grab from behind.

Uppercut Elbow Strike #4

The motion of this technique is similar to that of an uppercut punch. Use the forearm bone to strike upward at the jaw, throat, or chin. Make contact just below the tip of your striking elbow. You can also use it to attack the groin and abdomen when you are on the ground or lower than your opponent. Start in a right outlet stance. Bring the striking arm close to your body and thrust your elbow upward close to your front ear for proper follow-through. You may wish to keep your hand open to avoid striking yourself in the ear.

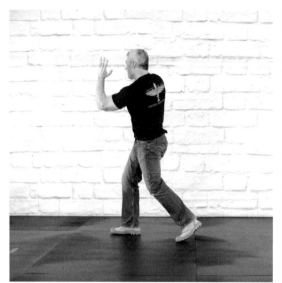 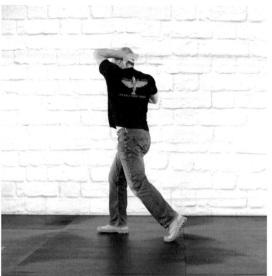

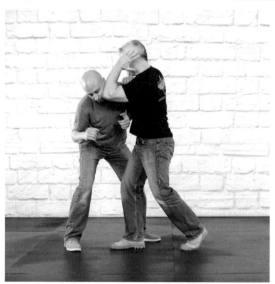

Uppercut elbow strike #4.

Vertical Elbow Drop Strike #5

The vertical elbow drop strike #5 is similar to the vertical hammer fist. Targets again include the back of the neck, the area between the shoulder blades, and the kidneys. If your opponent is on the ground, his face and groin can become targets. From your left outlet stance, execute the same body motion (a sudden drop) as with the vertical hammer fist, but this time connect with your elbow. Do not bring your arm higher than you would position it in your regular outlet stance. Make contact using the area just above the tip of your striking elbow. This elbow is particularly powerful and a natural fit following a straight knee strike. When the opponent doubles over, exposing the back of his neck and base of his skull, you can attack these vulnerable areas.

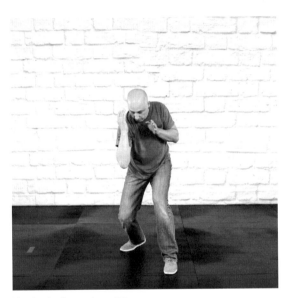

Vertical elbow drop #5.

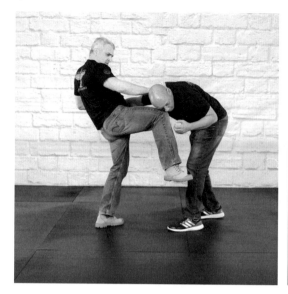 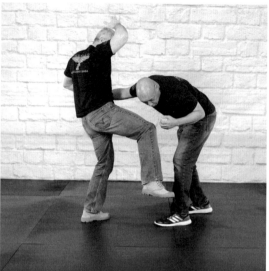

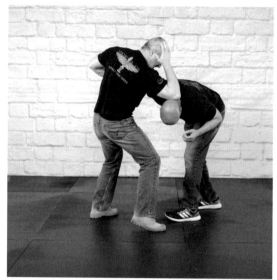

Vertical elbow drop #5 used with a knee-strike combination.

Rear Midsection Elbow Strike #6

The rear midsection elbow strike #6 delivers a compact strike to an opponent's groin, midsection, face, and other targets. In this strike, your hips once again create the power by opening up as you take a short step backward with the leg on the same side. Start in a regular left outlet stance. Keeping your striking arm close to your body, look over your shoulder in the direction of your strike. Step back slightly with the same-side leg as your striking arm. As you shift your body weight through the strike, make contact with the groin, using the area just above the tip of your striking elbow. You can either keep your hand open or clenched. The perpendicular rear elbow movement is readily applied to using a weapon (such as a pool cue, cane, umbrella or a rifle butt) to thrust behind you.

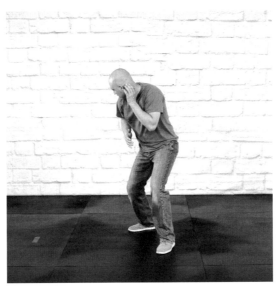

Rear midsection elbow strike #6.

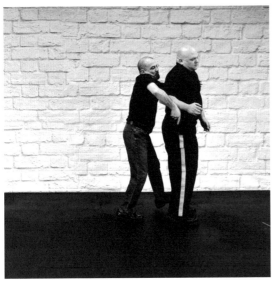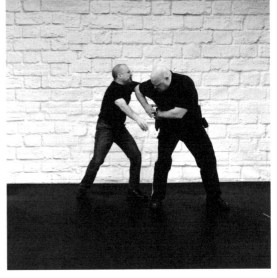

Rear midsection elbow strike #6 used in sidearm retention.

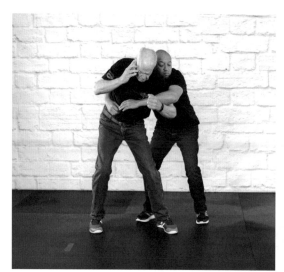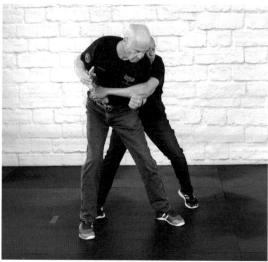

Rear midsection elbow strike #6 used in defending a rear bear-hug attempt.

Rear Vertical Elbow Strike #7

The rear vertical elbow strike #7 is another good follow-on to the short rear elbow. Start in the left outlet stance with your legs slightly bent. Make a strengthened, flexed hand or fist to strengthen your arms and shoulder. Look where you are striking. Then, explode upward with your hips, shoulder, and arm, targeting the solar plexus, throat, or face with your elbow. Make contact with the area just above the tip of your striking elbow. You can also use a blunt weapon with this strike.

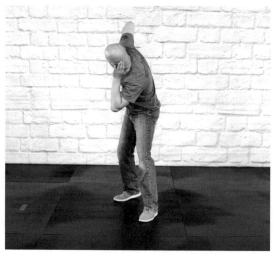

Rear vertical elbow strike #7.

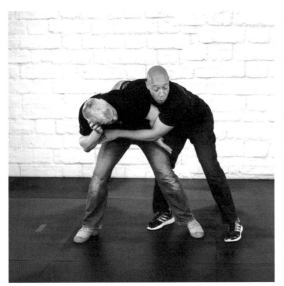 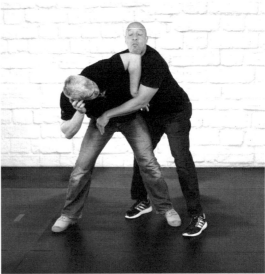

Rear vertical elbow strike #7 used in defending a rear bear-hug attempt.

Over-the-Top Elbow Strike #8

The over-the-top elbow strike #8 is designed to slam down on your opponent. Targets include the eye ridge, nose, ear, and throat. This can be combined strongly with horizontal and uppercut elbows into retzev. The over-the-top elbow uses a hip-pivot movement that's somewhere between those used in the straight punch and in the roundhouse punch. Beginning from your outlet stance, bring the striking elbow up and over, rotating over the top, or from head height to sternum. Make contact with the area just below the tip of your striking elbow. This strike can be especially effective if you are able to trap one or both of your opponent's arms with your lead arm to negate his defenses. You can also use a weapon to strike over the top; however, your arms should not cross. They should move in parallel instead. This over-the-top elbow is highly effective following a straight kick, which doubles the opponent over, exposing his temple and neck to attack.

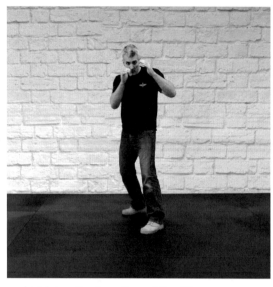 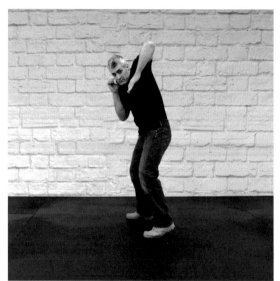

Lead over-the-top elbow strike #8.

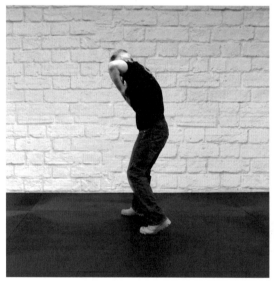 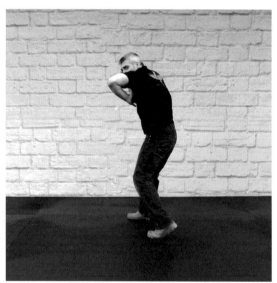

Lead over-the-top elbow strike #8. Note full front pivot.

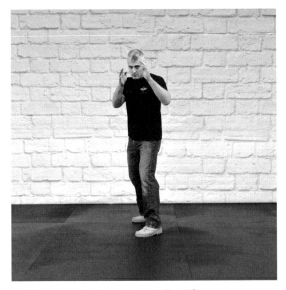 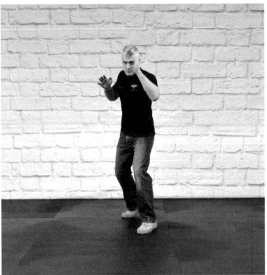

Rear over-the-top elbow strike #8.

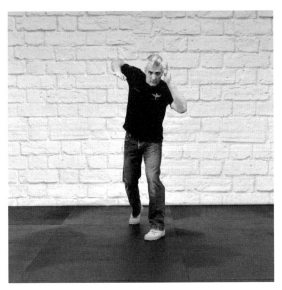 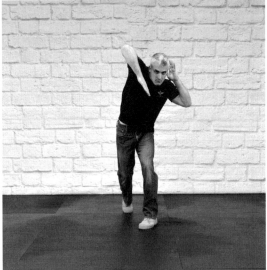

Rear over-the-top elbow strike #8.

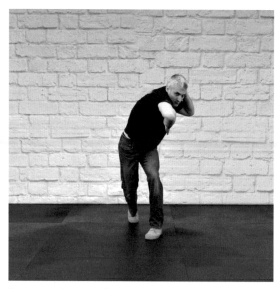

Rear over-the-top elbow strike #8. Note full rear pivot.

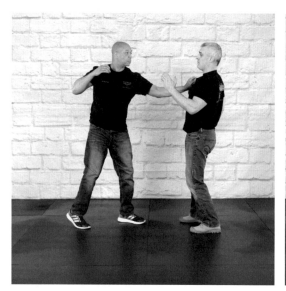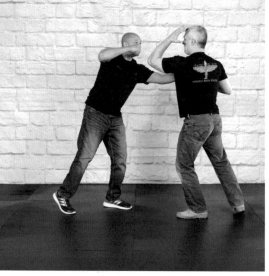

Rear over-the-top elbow strike #8 used in defending a combined shirt-grab and straight-punch attack.
Note: The gunt (angled elbow block) used to defend the straight punch is a modified #5 uppercut
elbow.

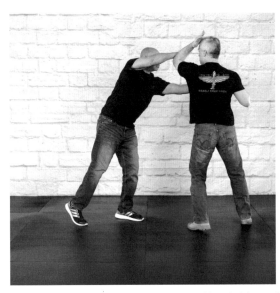

Rear over-the-top elbow strike #8 used in defending a combined shirt-grab and straight-punch attack. Note: The gunt (angled elbow block) used to defend the straight punch is a modified #5 uppercut elbow.

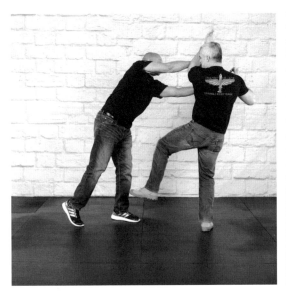 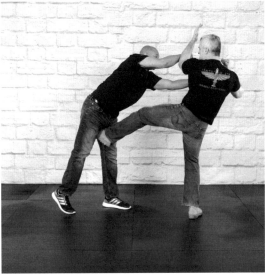

Rear over-the-top elbow strike #8 used in defending a combined shirt-grab and straight-punch attack.

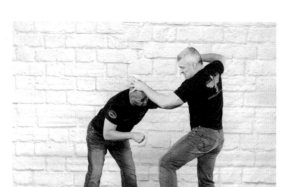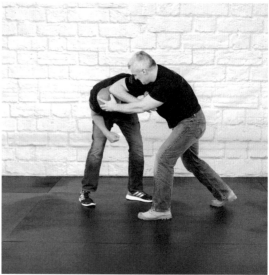

Rear over-the-top elbow strike #8 used in defending a combined shirt-grab and straight-punch attack.

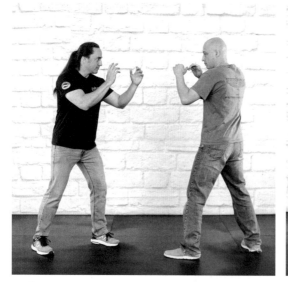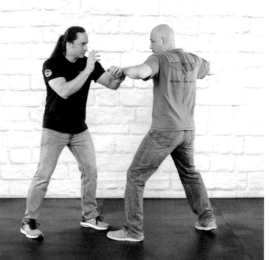

Rear over-the-top elbow strike #8 used in a lead arm-trap attack.

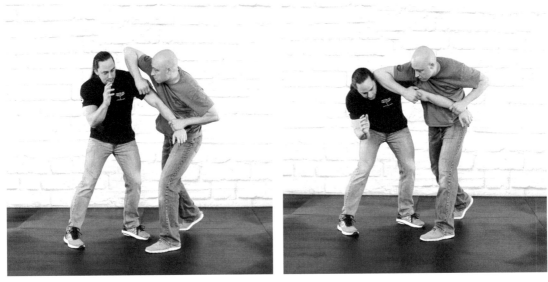

Rear over-the-top elbow strike #8 used in a lead arm-trap attack.

Forearm Elbow Strike #9

The forearm elbow strike #9 is a short, direct, and rapid strike. Aim for the throat, jaw, or nose. With your body weight behind it and with proper footwork, this technique is extremely powerful for knocking your opponent back, especially if you strike the throat. Stand in the left outlet stance with your hands in loose fists. Step forward with your left foot while lifting your left arm parallel to your chest, exposing the outer edge of your forearm. The upper- and lower-body movements are similar to those of the rear right straight punch, web strike, and knuckles punch, except for, of course, the striking area. Make contact with the ulna bone of your forearm. As your outer forearm extends to deliver the strike, tighten your fist, stepping forward to launch your full body weight through the strike. Make sure to step with both feet and thrust off the ball of the rear foot. Raise your left shoulder and tuck your chin to protect your jaw and neck. Keep your other hand up, protecting yourself, and be prepared to launch another combative. After striking to the throat, jaw, or nose, return to your left outlet stance.

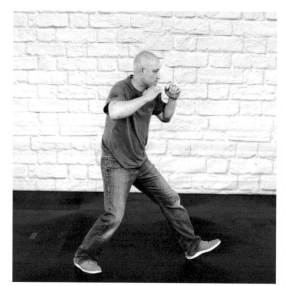 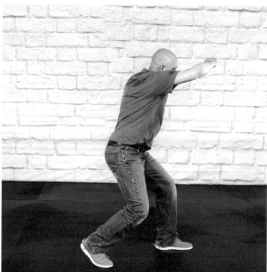

Forearm elbow strike #9.

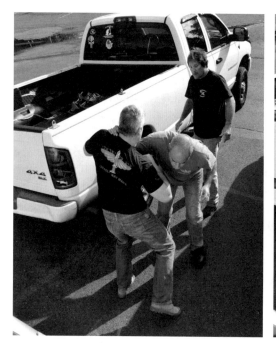 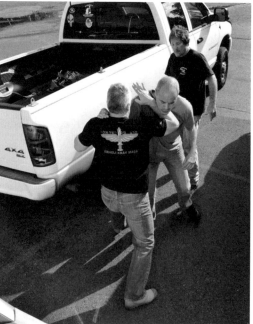

Forearm elbow strike #9 used in a multiple-opponent situation.

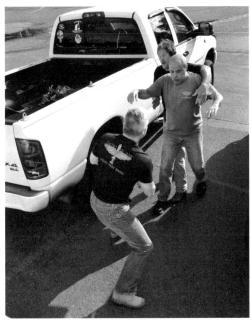

Forearm elbow strike #9 used in a multiple-opponent situation.

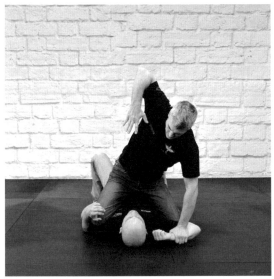
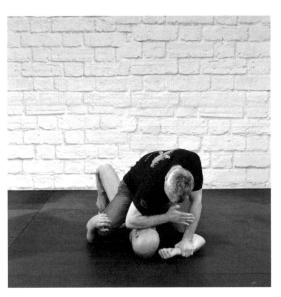

Forearm elbow strike #9 used in a mount.

Anti-Group Elbow Strike #10

The anti-group elbow strike #10 targets the jaw, throat, nose, and any other part of the face. This is employed when you must make your escape from multiple assailants. Look for a seam or opening between two opponents in a group confrontation and exploit the seam to make your escape. In krav maga, try never to put yourself between two assailants. If you can, flank one of the opponents to make your escape. Remember: always maneuver to the deadside, where you are behind the opponent's near shoulder or facing his back. However, if you must intentionally place yourself in this vulnerable position for a split second as you make your escape, this elbow variation reduces your vulnerability to attack.

The positioning of your arms is similar to throwing two simultaneous half-roundhouse punches—except, in this case, one fist is higher than the other. This is generally the left when beginning from the left outlet stance. The striking points are the first two knuckles on your fists and just below your elbow tips. This is so your fists do not collide if you make contact with both arms against opponents flanking you. Tuck your chin and bull your neck by raising your shoulders into your neck to protect from blows to the head. If necessary, your head can also serve as a modified battering ram. Once you are properly positioned, run and burst through your opponents to safety. This technique can be practiced with two partners holding two kicking shields high and away from their bodies. Target pads may also be used; however, kicking shields provide a larger target and additional safety for your partners.

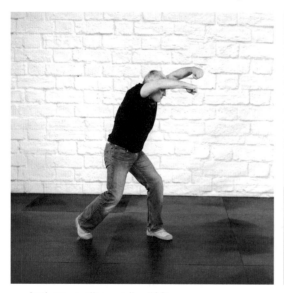 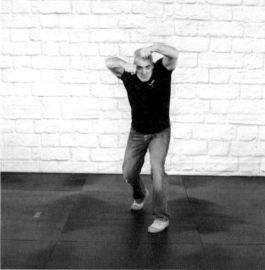

Anti-group elbow strike #10.

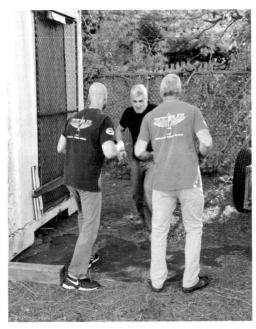

Anti-group elbow strike #10 used to escape when there is no choice but to split the opponents.

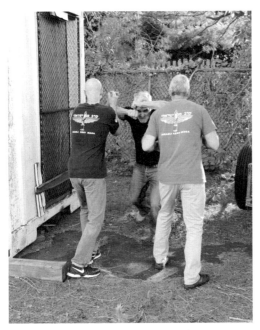 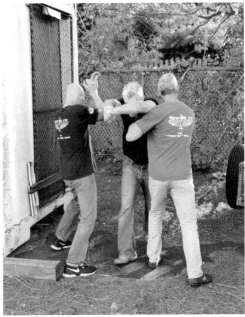

Anti-group elbow strike #10 used to escape when there is no choice but to split the opponents.

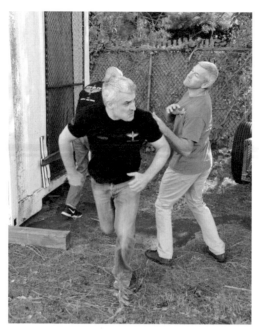

Anti-group elbow strike #10 used to escape when there is no choice but to split the opponents.

Combative Family #5: Hooks, Horizontal Palm-Heel Strikes, and Chops

Lead Hook Punch

Hook punches are powerful and can circumvent an opponent's defense. The punch's path usually follows whatever opening or vulnerability your opponent gives you. Targets usually include the jaw, cheek, throat, and ear. A note of caution: The mastoid behind the ear is dense bone, and this target can damage your hand. Begin in your regular outlet stance with your hands protecting your face. Connect with your target with your lead arm parallel to the ground, with the elbow bent at 90 degrees or slightly more. Make contact with the first two knuckles, your palm facing the ground. As you deliver the hook, pivot on your lead foot in the same direction as the punch so your lead heel nearly faces your target. As you pivot your heel, turn the rest of your body, but keep your eyes on the target. Adjust your rear foot slightly to accommodate your lead foot's movement. Keep your rear hand up in a fighting position. You can also try punching with your pinkie down and thumb up. Although physiology dictates that you'll punch with less power, because your deltoids and other shoulder muscles are not as actively involved, some practitioners prefer the "knuckles up" roundhouse punch because they feel the shoulder group is stronger. In addition, this hand position offers some additional protection to your exposed ribs.

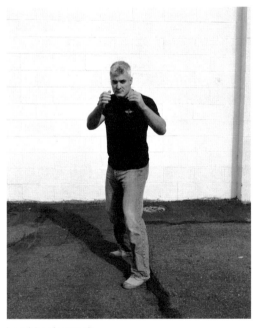

Lead hook punch.

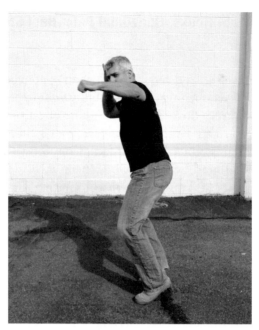

Lead hook punch. Note full pivot for full reach extension and power just prior to clenching the fist for impact.

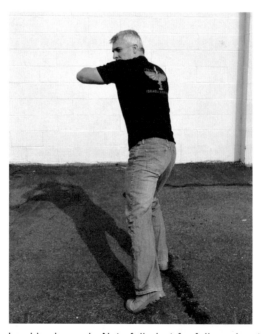

Lead hook punch. Note full pivot for full reach extension and power.

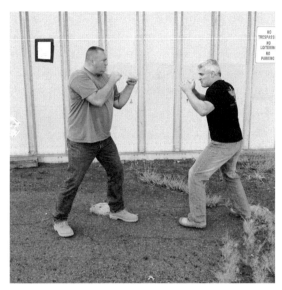

Lead hook punch to circumvent an opponent's defense.

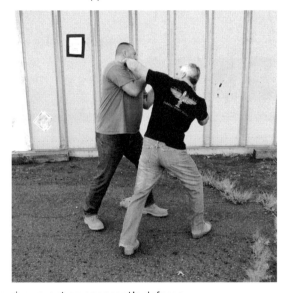

Lead hook punch to circumvent an opponent's defense.

Rear Hook Punch

Similar in movement to the lead hook punch, you'll deliver the rear hook punch instead with your rear arm. Begin in your regular outlet stance with your hands protecting your face. As you deliver a rear hook punch with your rear fist, pivot your core in the same direction as the punch. This will increase the power of the strike. At the same time, move the lead foot in the same direction to accommodate the rear foot's movement. Connect with your target with your lead arm parallel to the ground, with the elbow bent at 90 degrees or slightly more than 90 degrees. Make contact with the first two knuckles, your palm facing the ground. Keep your chin tucked.

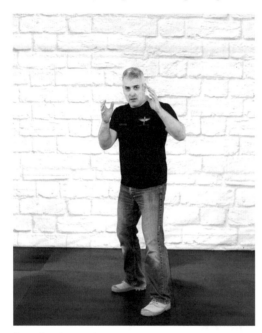 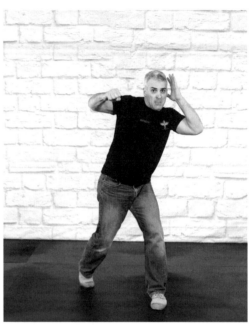

Rear hook punch.

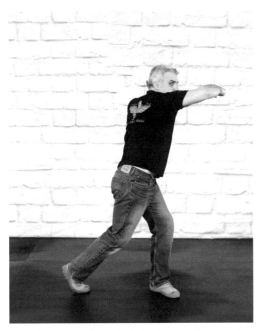

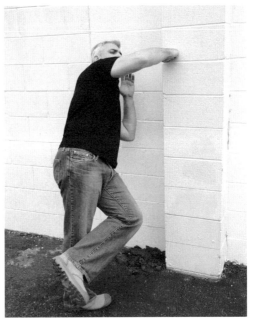

Rear hook punch. Note full pivot for full reach extension and power.

Rear hook-punch wrist alignment.

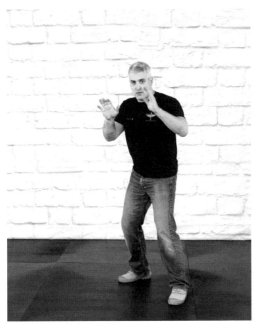

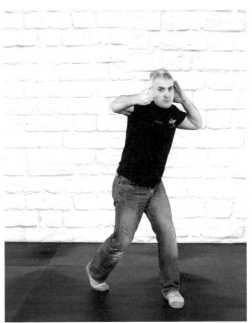

Rear hook punch, inverted-fist option.

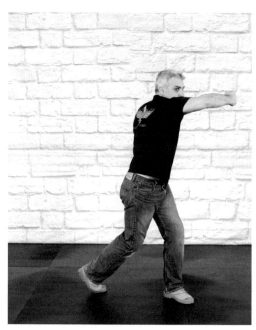

Rear hook punch, inverted-fist option. Note full pivot for full reach extension and power.

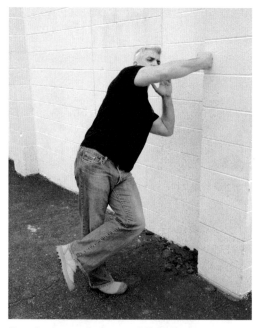

Rear hook punch, inverted-fist alignment.

Lead-Rear Hook Punch Combination (Not Depicted)

This "one-two" hook punch combination, while not depicted, is represented in the left-right horizontal elbow strike #1 combination photos. This one-two lead-rear hook punch combination takes advantage of the momentum of your body. Begin in your regular outlet stance with your hands protecting your face. Deliver a lead roundhouse strike. Then immediately follow up with a rear roundhouse punch.

A note on hook punches: I personally prefer using palm-heel strikes rather than hook punches because of the vulnerability of the hand when orchestrating a hook punch. Do not think that the hook punch is not a powerful knockdown combative, because it is. My personal preference is simply not to rely heavily on hook punches (and uppercut punches). From a teaching aspect, I think it is easier for students to learn the horizontal palm-heel strike. Of equal note, for professional training, a closed-fist punch to a Kevlar helmet is likely to damage your hand, whereas a palm-heel strike likely will not. (The palm-heel strike can still rattle the head, even when protected with a helmet.)

Body Hook Shot

The body hook shot combative delivers a roundhouse punch to the torso, primarily targeting the kidneys, liver, and floating ribs. Perform the same lower-body and hip movements as in the lead and rear high roundhouses, but change your hand position into an inverted punch, keeping your elbow in close to your torso and your forearm parallel to the ground. You can combine high and low roundhouse punches to form a devastating attack. Follow up with a lead high punch, and then a rear low punch—or vice versa. In addition, you can throw a high-low or low-high combination with the same-side arm.

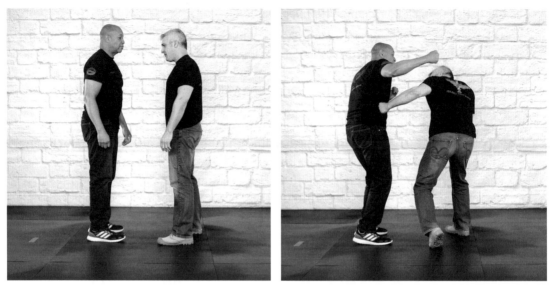

Body hook shot used to preempt a hook-punch attack. Note full pivot for full reach extension and power.

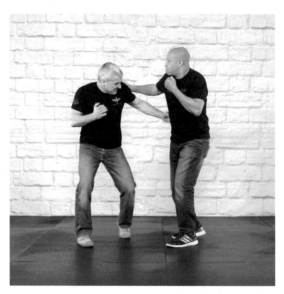

Body hook shot used to preempt a hook-punch attack, opposite angle. Note full pivot for full reach extension and power.

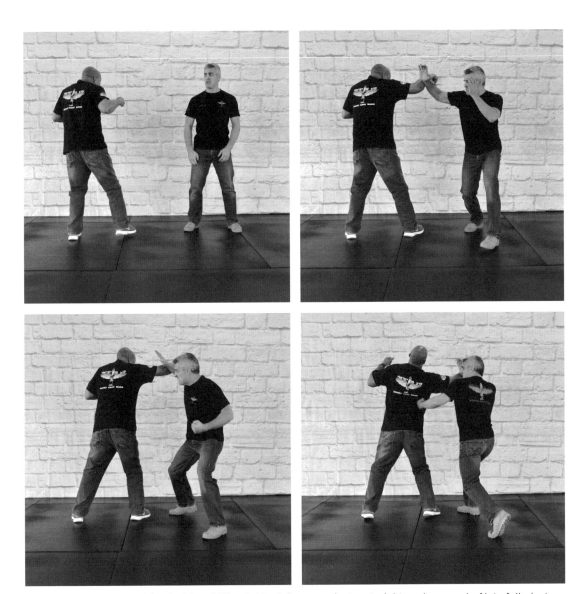

Body hook shot combined with a 360 outside defense against a straight sucker punch. Note full pivot for full reach extension and power.

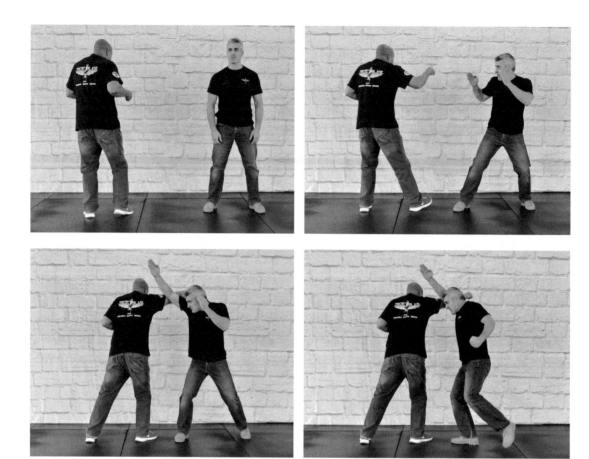

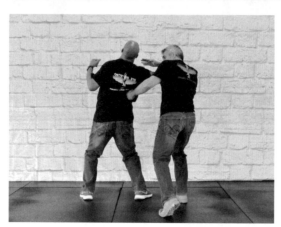

Body hook shot combined with a stabbing, sliding defense against a straight sucker punch. Note full pivot for full reach extension and power.

Body Shovel Punch

The body shovel punch targets the stomach or internal organs. The hip rotation is similar to that of a straight punch. Wrist alignment is also similar to that of the straight punch and is formed by simply inverting the wrist. A slight bend upward stabilizes the wrist. Contact is made with the first two knuckles. An advanced version of the punch twists the wrist slightly after impact to the body to increase the damage.

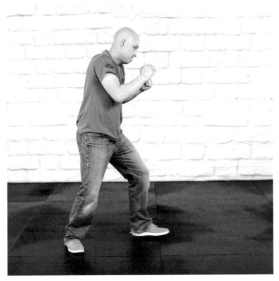
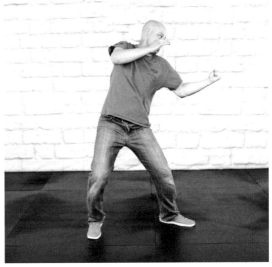

Lead body shovel punch.

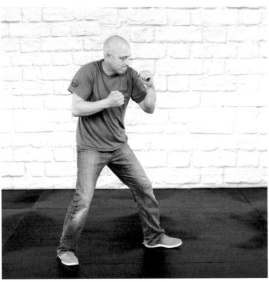
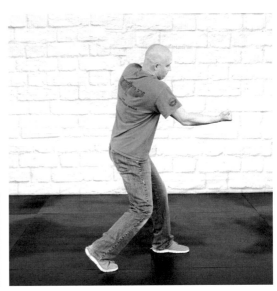

Rear body shovel punch.

Uppercut Punch

The uppercut punch can seriously damage your opponent's exposed chin, throat, or groin—the last target especially when you are on your knees and your opponent is standing. This strike is thrown from a dynamic-movement stance, which is the outlet stance in motion. Bend your knees slightly to generate power from the lower body, allowing your hips to explode through the target. For the lead uppercut punch, pivot the lead leg inward and straighten your knees as you punch, delivering an upward blow. A common mistake is to drop the arm rather than the body. Be sure to align the wrist properly, as this strike places considerable pressure on the wrist when you hit bone. Deliver the rear uppercut punch the same way, except pivot the rear foot inward. Make contact with the first two knuckles, turning your fist toward the opponent, so the palm is facing inward toward you. (See also the following takedown defense: rear knee against a takedown attempt combined with an uppercut punch.)

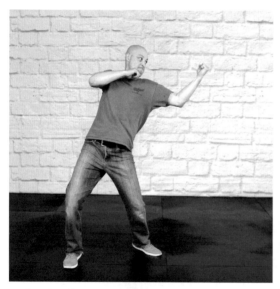 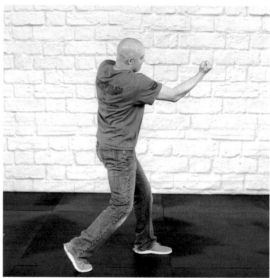

Lead and rear uppercut punches.

Horizontal Palm-Heel Strike

The lead horizontal palm-heel strike is a highly effective strike to the temple, ears, and jaw. This strike is particularly useful, as it uses an open hand, thereby minimizing the danger to your knuckles and wrist. In addition, the strike can (and should) be delivered without telegraphing, making it more difficult to spot and, thus, defend. As previously noted, I prefer the horizontal palm-heel strike (and chops, described in the next technique) instead of hook-punch combatives.

Begin in your regular left outlet stance with your hands protecting your face. As you deliver the horizontal palm-heel strike, pivot on the balls of both feet in the same direction as the strike. This will increase the power of the strike as your lower body and hips move in tandem with your torso and shoulder to generate power. Strike with the lower fleshy portion of your hand at the desired target area. Keep your other hand up, protecting yourself, and be prepared to launch another combative. The correct way to deliver the horizontal palm-heel strike is to keep your forearm and hand partially tense just prior to impact, when you will then strengthen the entire arm and hand.

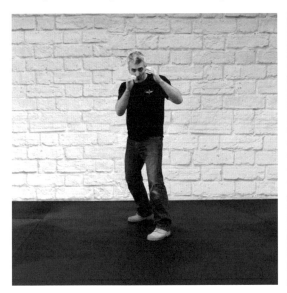 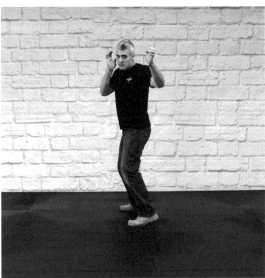

Lead horizontal palm-heel strike.

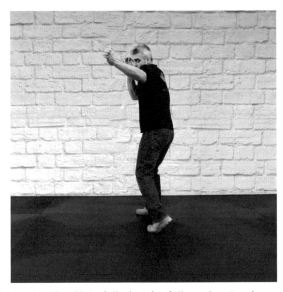

Lead horizontal palm-heel strike. Note full pivot for full reach extension and power.

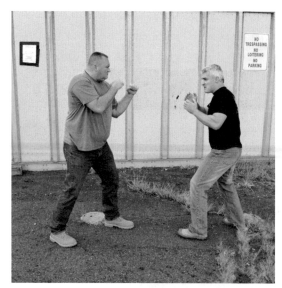 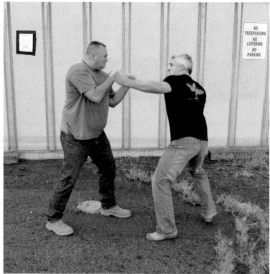

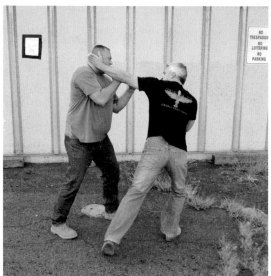

Lead horizontal palm-heel strike used to circumvent an opponent's defense. Note full pivot for full reach extension and power.

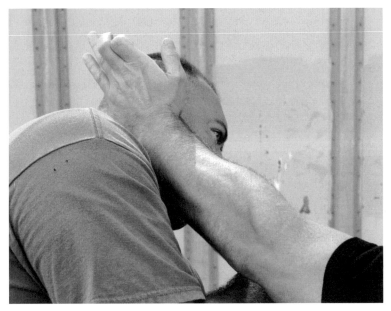

Lead horizontal palm-heel strike, impact close-up.

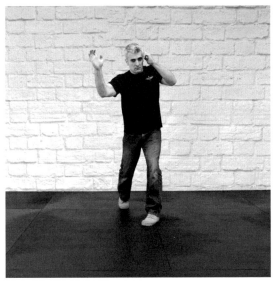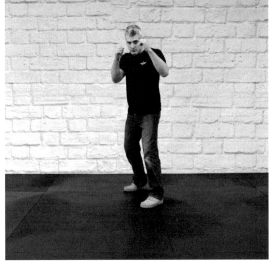

Rear horizontal palm-heel strike.

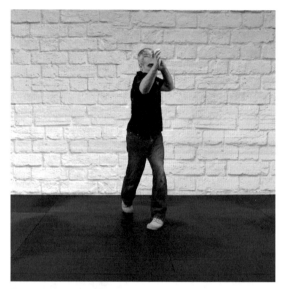

Rear horizontal palm-heel strike. Note full pivot for full reach extension and power.

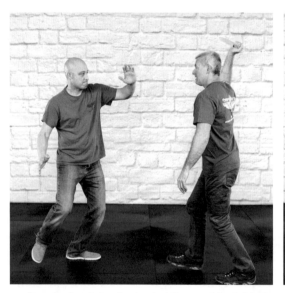
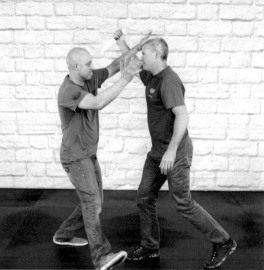

Rear horizontal palm-heel strike used in defending an overhead knife-attack ambush.

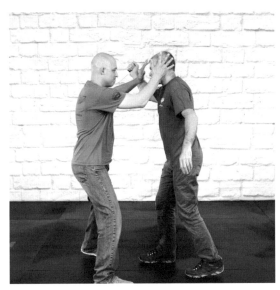

Rear horizontal palm-heel strike used in defending an overhead knife-attack ambush.

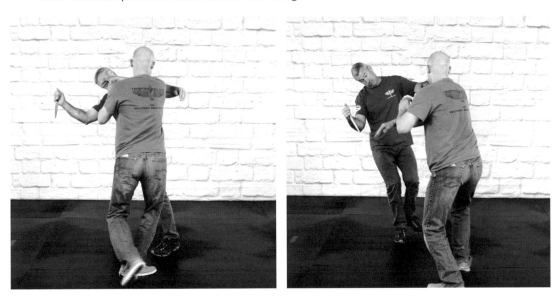

Rear horizontal palm-heel strike used in initially defending an overhead knife-attack ambush. Note full pivot for full reach extension and power. Note, as depicted, this is only a partial defense. The defender could flee or reengage to disarm the attacker as opportune.

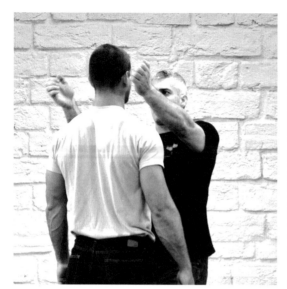 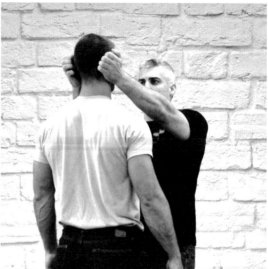

Horizontal double palm-heel strikes.

Inside and Outside Chops

The chop is a strong combative that can be utilized on whatever opening your opponent gives you, especially the carotid artery, windpipe, throat, neck, and nose. It may also be employed to target internal organs such as the kidneys, spleen, and liver. There are two basic types of chops: (1) inside chops and (2) outside chops.

When delivering the strike, be sure to position the hand correctly to avoid injuring it. Poor technique could mean breaking your pinkie finger. For either an inside or outside chop, contact is made with the fleshy part of your hand (the *triquetrum* and lunate bones), just below where the hand joins the wrist on the pinkie side of your hand. Use a chop-like motion to stun and injure your opponent. Note: You may also use the forearm to attack the neck should the distance be too short to execute a chop. To deliver maximum power and reach, as with your hook punches and horizontal palm-heel strikes, pivot correctly on your feet to engage the hips, placing your body mass behind the strike.

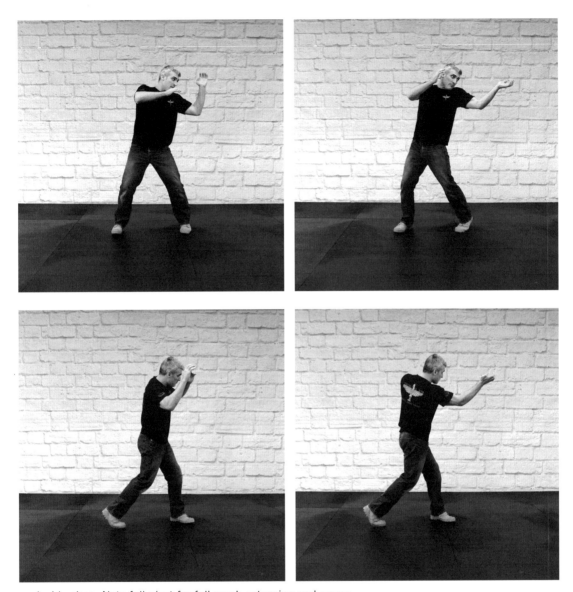

Inside chop. Note full pivot for full reach extension and power.

Inside Chop

To deliver an inside chop, strike with your rear arm, keeping your elbow close to your side and bent approximately 45 degrees. Begin in your regular left outlet stance with your hands protecting your face. As you deliver the rear chop, pivot on the balls of both feet in the same direction as the chop. This will increase the power of the strike, as your lower body and hips move in tandem with your torso and shoulder to generate power. Your wrist will fold back, so contact is made with the lower "knife" edge, or the fleshy underside, of the palm and bone just below the wrist joint. The positioning resembles the knuckles-edge strike to the throat, except the wrist is slightly turned out. Keep your other hand up, protecting yourself, and be prepared to launch another combative. The correct way to chop is to keep your forearm and hand partially tense just prior to impact, when you will then strengthen the entire arm and hand.

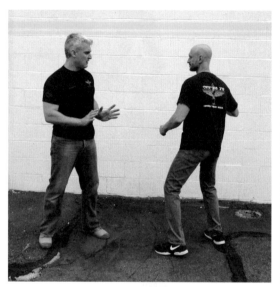 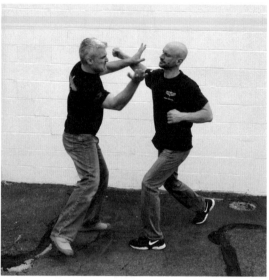

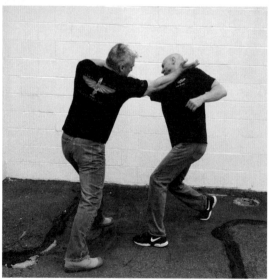

Inside chop combined with an outside 360 defense in defending a hook punch. Note full pivot for full reach extension and power.

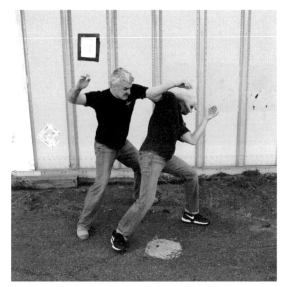 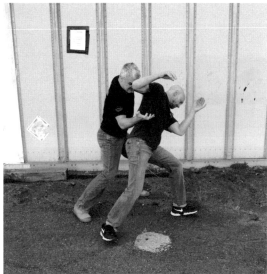

Inside chop targeting the ribs.

Outside Chop

The outside chop best targets the sides of the neck (carotid arteries), throat, and nose. The outside chop uses the same striking surface as the inward chop; however, the wrist is not bent, and the hand and forearm are in straight alignment. As you deliver the chop, you will pivot the lead foot in the same direction as the strike, so your toes turn past the target. Pivot on the ball of your foot and turn the rest of your body, but keep your eyes on the target. Adjust your rear foot slightly to accommodate the movement of your lead foot. Keep your rear hand up in a fighting position. The same partially tense movement applies as with the inward chop, until the hand is fully strengthened at the moment before impact. The outside chop is also useful because it keeps a brace between you and your opponent to prevent him from slipping behind you to take your back for a take-down or throw.

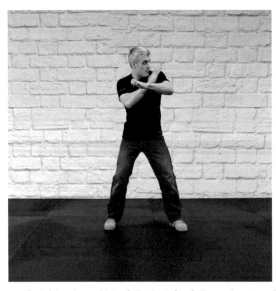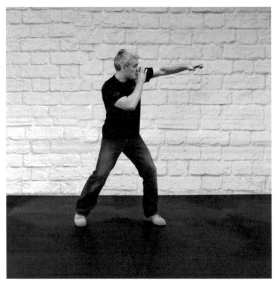

Outside chop. Note full pivot for full reach extension and power.

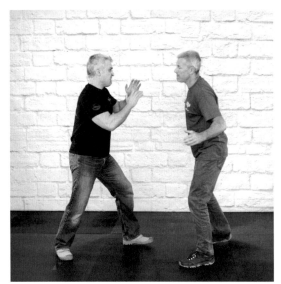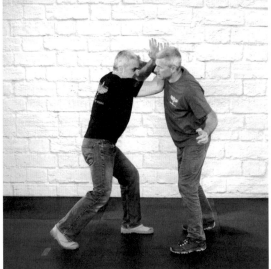

Outside chop combined with a double arm interception in defending a hook punch.

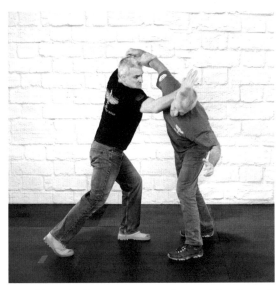

Outside chop combined with a double-arm interception in defending a hook punch. Note full pivot for full reach extension and power.

"Clothesline" Arimi Strike

The "clothesline" *arimi* strike is a powerful forearm strike targeting the opponent's throat, neck, or nose. The footwork is similar to that of a straight punch or elbow #9 forearm strike. Contact is made with your radial bone, usually against the opponent's throat or neck. Keep a slight bend in your elbow to prevent hyperextension upon contact. Note: The arimi strike can easily facilitate a standing-choke option, if you continue from the initial strike to wrap your arm around the opponent's neck.

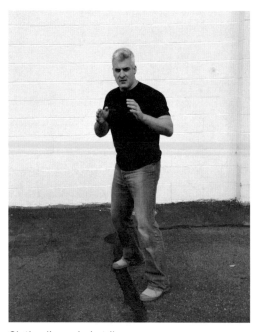 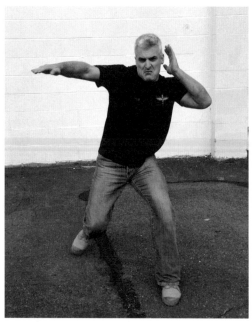

Clothesline arimi strike.

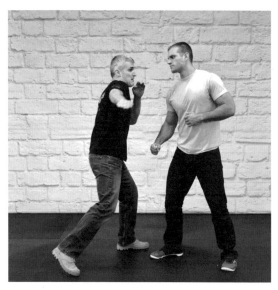 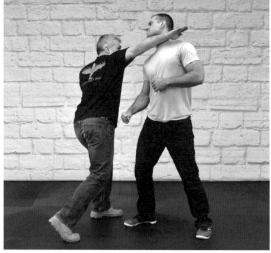

Clothesline arimi strike.

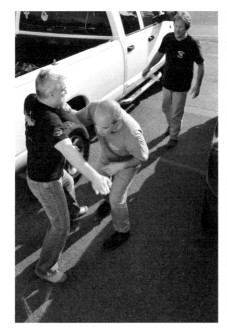 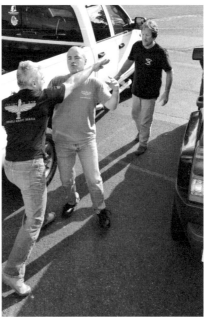

Clothesline arimi strike used in a multiple-opponent situation.

Rear Straight Forearm Strike or Hammer Fist

The rear straight forearm strike or hammer fist targets the nose, jaw, or throat. Stand in a left outlet stance with your hands in loose fists. Look at the opponent a fraction of a second before you commence the strike; this way your head will lead the body. Pivot your right leg slightly onto the ball of the foot as you drive your hips, rear shoulder, and outer forearm through your target. Tuck your chin into your right shoulder to protect it from an incoming attack. Keep your left hand up to protect yourself, and be prepared to launch another combative. Note: The way you turn your head and pivot the lower body in this technique is the same as with rear horizontal elbow strike #3.

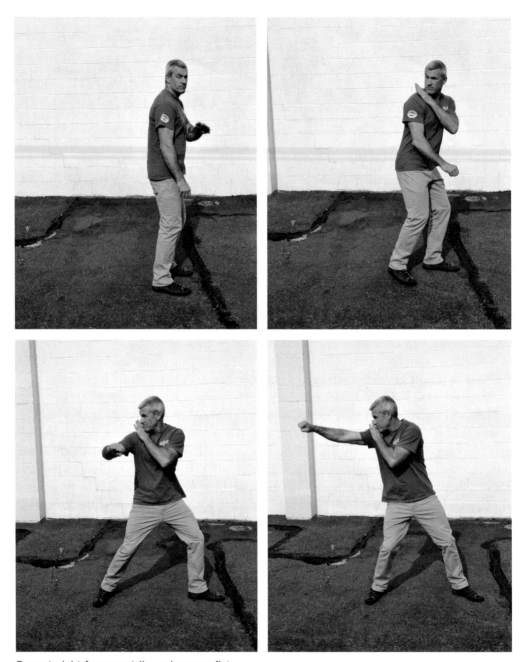

Rear straight forearm strike or hammer fist.

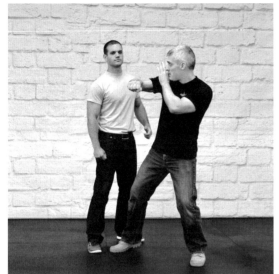 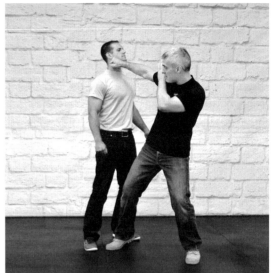

Rear straight forearm strike or hammer fist.

Combatives Family #6: Headbutts and Biting

Headbutts

The headbutt can be a highly effective counterattack, especially when you smash your opponent's face by surprise. A note of caution, however: some defenders may not have the neck strength to sustain delivering a headbutt, so this tactic may not be suitable for everyone. Krav maga incorporates both lead and rear headbutts.

Front Headbutt

The front headbutt is delivered by bulling the neck and preparing the neck for contact, which is made using the thickest part of the skull, the crown. The entire body is used in the front-headbutt combative; you do not just bring back the head to deliver the strike. This combative could be used in a grab or bear-hug situation where your arms are pinned or not free. Targets include the opponent's temple, chin, and nose. Be careful not to strike your opponent's teeth, for the obvious reasons of injury to your head and possible transmission of pathogens through lacerated skin.

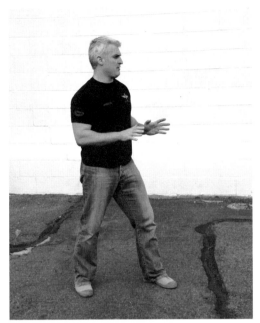 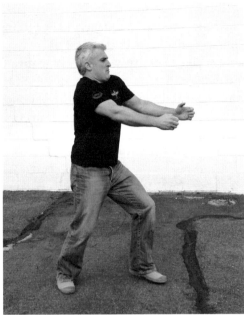

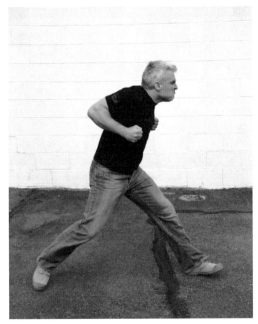

Front headbutt.

Rear Headbutt

The rear headbutt is delivered by bulling the neck and preparing the neck for contact. Contact is made using the back of the skull. Once again, the entire body is used in the rear-headbutt combative. This combative could be used when defending against a rear bear hug or in certain weapon-defense situations when the assailant is threatening you from the rear. Targets include the opponent's temple, chin, and nose. Again, try not to strike his teeth for the obvious reasons of injury to your head and possible transmission of pathogens through lacerated skin.

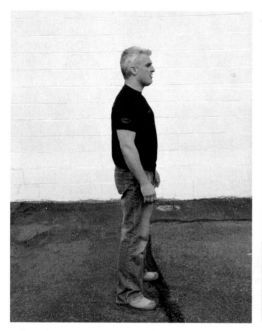 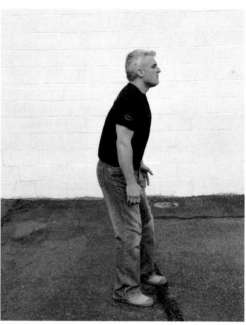

Rear headbutt.

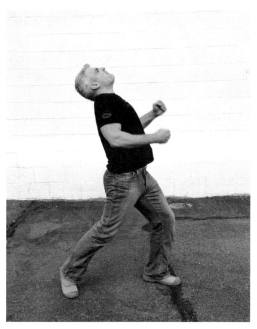

Rear headbutt.

Biting

Biting is a primordial, highly effective, visceral, and animalistic tactic. This combative is usually used as a last resort when other defenses have failed. Accordingly, concerns about communicable diseases are set aside to prioritize surviving the situation. Many combat-oriented movies depict biting in such circumstances. For optimum effect, cant your head and use your incisors to tear the attacker's flesh. Biting may be the default tactic when you are choked or grabbed in such a way that no other combative is available. Remember: the krav maga curriculum emphasizes using whatever means are at your disposal to defeat an attack. Usually an attacker's arm or hand is somewhere near your face, but, as another example, if you are caught in an armbar, you may have to bite into the attacker's Achilles tendon to keep your arm from being broken. Here a few scenarios and examples where your teeth may have to come into play:

- An attacker is choking you from the rear, and you cannot lever his arm free, but your mouth is close to his arm.
- An attacker is choking you from the rear with an implement (such as a baseball bat), and you are on the ground in position to bite his arm or hand holding the implement.
- An attacker has your arms pinned in a bear hug from the front and is lifting you up.

- You are on the ground, fighting for your life, and some part of the attacker's body is close to your mouth.

- You are part of a group trying to wrest an edged weapon away from an assailant. Your job is to get him to drop the weapon: bite his hand or mouth.

Always keep in mind that an attacker can also bite you from an infighting or ground position.

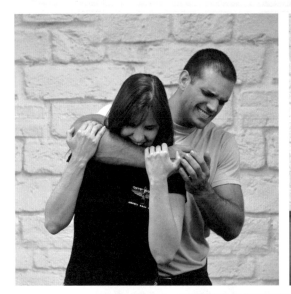
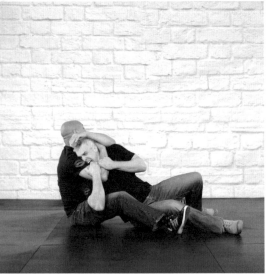

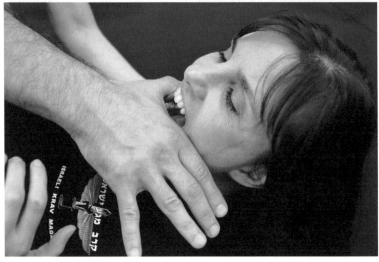

Biting.

Combatives Family #7: Choke Holds

Choke Holds

Chokes must only be used in a self-defense situation where you have an acute and genuine fear that the attacker intends you serious bodily harm. In krav maga parlance, there are two types of choke holds: air chokes and blood chokes. Both techniques achieve the same result: unconsciousness, brain damage, or death, depending on the force and length of time the choke is applied. Chokes are fight enders.

Air chokes cut off the oxygen supply to the brain by preventing air from refilling the lungs. In addition, a choke can cause severe damage to the trachea, hyoid bone, and larynx. The tongue can also become lodged in the back of the throat and occlude airflow. Be aware that a choke or strangulation technique can exacerbate or trigger a preexisting medical condition, possibly resulting in death.

Blood chokes or strangulation techniques stop the flow of blood by constricting the carotid artery and jugular veins on the sides of the neck. These veins carry oxygenated and deoxygenated blood. Do not allow anyone to get his or her hands, arms, or legs around your neck. Choke techniques can utilize the hands, forearms, or other objects such as a stick or rolled-up magazine placed across the throat. The key to proper chokes is using your hands and arms to provide leverage and compression that leave your adversary few, if any, defenses. The narrower the choking implement, the easier the insertion under the adversary's chin to apply the choke. The ulnar and radial edges of the wrist and forearm are particularly well suited to apply compression to the throat and neck. An adversary's clothing can be used against him, and so can yours against you—so beware. Keep your head close to your adversary to avoid countertechniques. The three techniques below are applied from the rear, the most advantageous choking position.

NOTE: CHOKES ARE EXTREMELY DANGEROUS FOR USE AS COMBATIVES. YOU MAY NOT RECOGNIZE OR KNOW WHEN YOU HAVE RENDERED SOMEONE TEMPORARILY UNCONSCIOUS. IF YOU CONTINUE TO APPLY THE CHOKE, YOU RISK KILLING THE OPPONENT.

An opponent may tuck his chin or shrug his shoulders in a preliminary defense. This initial defense, however, can easily be defeated by yanking back on the opponent's philtrum (the vertical groove on the upper lip), penetrating eye sockets, or attacking other susceptible pressure points to lift his chin, exposing his throat.

You should use three people when practicing choke holds: two to drill and the third to monitor the situation. This will ensure the person applying the technique stops at the instant the choke is successfully applied or at the first sign of danger. When practicing with a partner, take the utmost care. When allowing yourself to be choked, you will not be able to speak if the choke is properly applied. Have a prearranged signal that consists of "tapping" your partner to tell him to immediately release the choke.

Forearm-Blade Choke

The forearm-blade choke applies crushing pressure to the opponent's windpipe, depriving his brain of oxygen by the pressure of the radius or blade of the forearm. This pressure can collapse and crush the windpipe. Keep your body tight to your opponent and tuck your head. Clasp your nonchoking arm with your hand and pull your forearm into you. When practicing with a partner, use extreme caution.

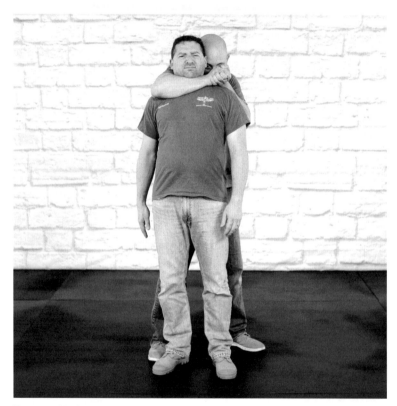

Forearm-blade choke.

Crook-of-the-Elbow Choke

The crook-of-the-elbow choke or "V choke" applies pressure to the opponent's carotid sheath on both sides of the neck, occluding blood flow to his brain. Pressure is applied using your biceps muscle and radius of the arm. Keep your body tight to your opponent with your head tucked. Clasp your right hand with your left hand and squeeze your arms together to constrict blood flow. When practicing with a partner, use extreme caution.

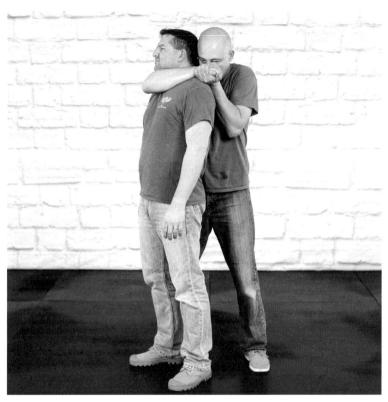

Crook-of-the-elbow choke.

Professional Rear Naked Choke

The professional rear naked choke can be thought of as a superior combination of the two previous choking techniques because of the extreme pressure that may be applied. The blade of the forearm and biceps apply pressure to the opponent's carotid sheath on both sides of the neck, stopping blood flow to his brain. For a right-arm professional rear naked choke, grab your left biceps muscle with your right hand (or jam your right fist into the crook of your left arm). Your nonchoking arm will snake behind your opponent's head, and your hand will be placed on the rear of his skull. Do not place the hand too high because a defender can remove or pluck it away to disable the choke.

To apply pressure, squeeze your choking arm toward you and the biceps of your nonchoking arm. At the same time, exert pressure forward with your cupped hand, and lean the side of your head into your hand for added choking pressure. Clasp your hand with your nonchoking arm and squeeze your arms together to constrict blood flow. Your body is essentially both leaning forward (on the top plane, which is your left arm's radial bone) and pulling back (on the bottom plane, which is your right arm's radial bone) to exert maximum choking pressure. Keep your body tight to your opponent while tucking your head. Keep your hips square to his. To optimize the choke, you may rock the assailant slightly to one side and then the other to cinch the choke and thwart his counters. The examples depicted show a defense against a hook punch where the defender counterattacks with a counterpunch to the attacker's head and then spins the attacker into a rear naked professional choke. When on the ground, do not cross your ankles (creating "hooks") unless you can obtain a "figure-4" position and can keep your legs on your opponent's thighs to prevent him from applying ankle locks. This choke—both standing or on the ground—is highly effective.

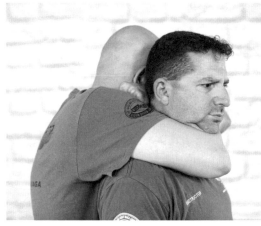
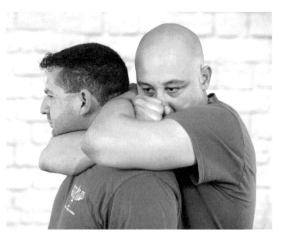

Professional rear naked choke, opposite views.

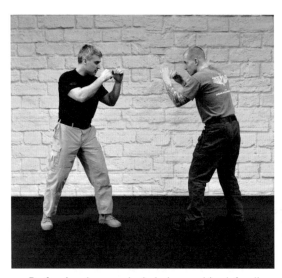
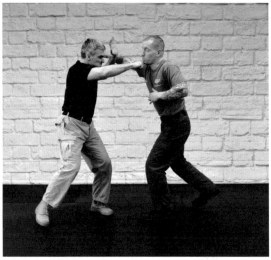

Professional rear naked choke used in defending a hook punch.

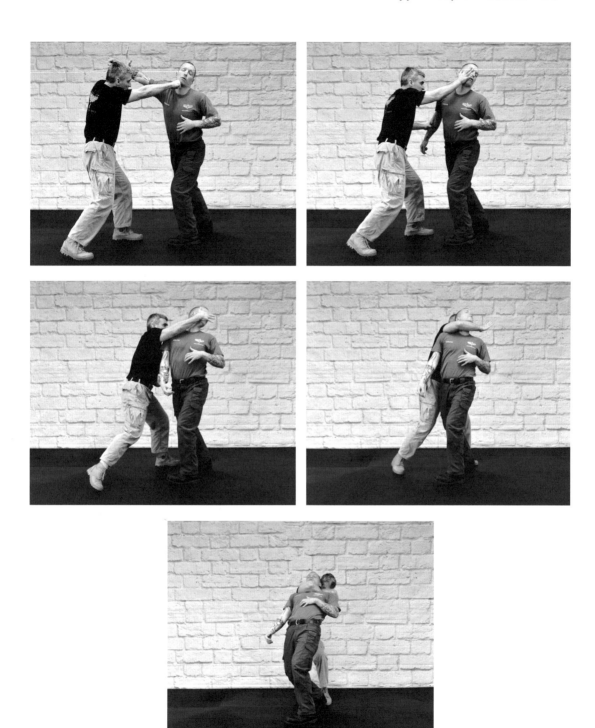

Professional rear naked choke used in defending a hook punch.

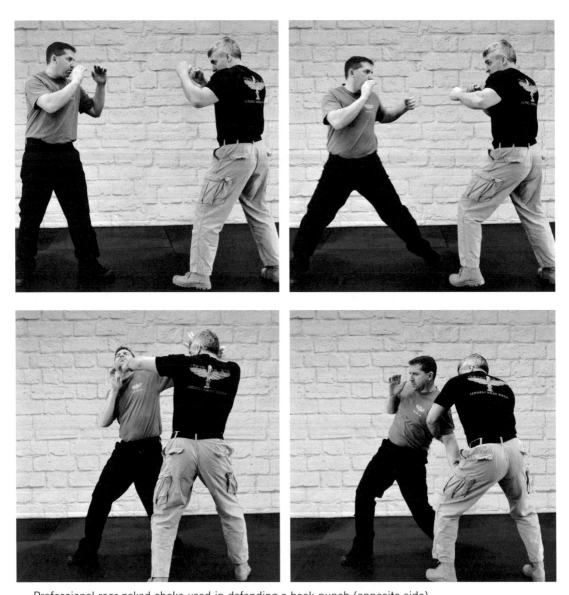

Professional rear naked choke used in defending a hook punch (opposite side).

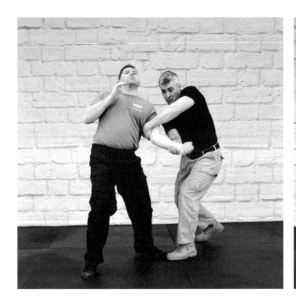 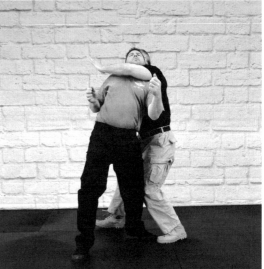

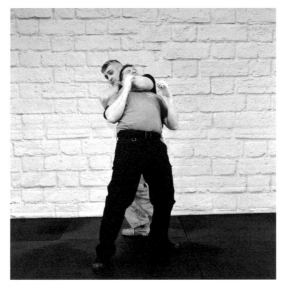

Professional rear naked choke used in defending a hook punch (opposite side).

Bonus Technique: Rear Naked Choke Defense Variation Using Rear Straight-Knee Counterattack

Forearm chokes and "professional chokes" from the rear are some of the most effective and dangerous strangulation techniques. Due to the popularity of MMA, even untrained people have learned to put a rear naked choke in action. This choke can crush your windpipe or cut off the blood flow from the carotid arteries to the brain. These are powerful chokes because the attacker's entire body can be maneuvered to exert maximum force. This tactic is covered in chapter 3, "Upper-Body Combatives."

You must react instantaneously to these highly effective offensive techniques. This technique variation takes into account that, as noted, 85 percent or more of the world's population is right-side dominant. Therefore, an attacker is most likely to choke you with his right arm, using his left arm to support the choke. Our goal in using this highly effective variation is to turn against the choke one way and one way only. You don't have a decision to make whether to turn to your left or your right; you are simply always going to turn to your left. The key to success with this defense—and any type of rear choke or grab defense—is tactile feel training: as soon as you feel an arm choking or grabbing you, react instantaneously and instinctively (always the goal of all krav maga training) by breaking the grip and choke angle followed by a near-simultaneous straight knee to the groin.

Note: If you cannot release immediately from the blood choke from the rear, revert to a modified side-headlock release, but do not release your arms from the attacker's forearm until you can breathe enough to execute the side-headlock release. This modified release keeps your inside (left) arm exerting as much pressure as you can on the attacker's forearm under your chin. While keeping pressure on your attacker's choking arm with your initial defense, turn into the attacker with your outside (right) leg and deliver multiple attacks to the attacker's groin. Once you have "loosened up" your attacker, you have the option of your regular side-headlock release.

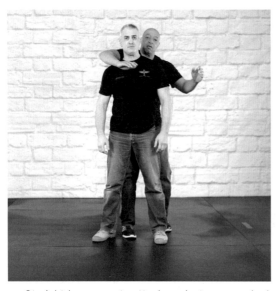 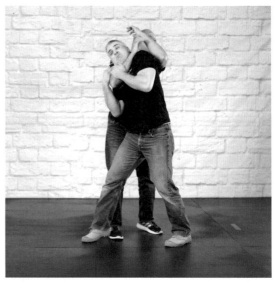

Straight-knee counterattack against a rear naked choke attempt.

As soon as you feel the attacker trying to wrap his arm around your neck, tuck your chin down and turn sharply away to your right while simultaneously raising your arms to catch the attacker's elbow crook or forearm. Importantly (and ideally), you accomplish this initial defense before the attacker can clasp his hands or secure both his arms together. Yank down with both your arms to forcefully clear the attacker's arm from your chin and neck area.

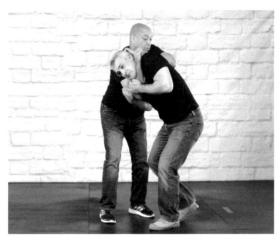

Straight-knee counterattack against a rear naked choke attempt.

As you create separation, dip your right shoulder and step slightly backward and fully across the attacker's front with your right leg while wheeling your right shoulder across the attacker's front. You may be able to deliver a right shoulder-smash attack into the attacker's midsection if your timing is good.

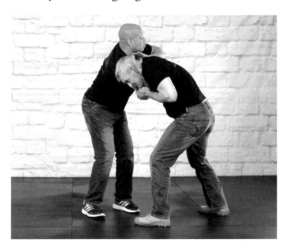

Straight-knee counterattack against a rear naked choke attempt.

Continue to step through and underneath the attacker's right armpit while holding the attacker's arm firmly pinned against your body with both your arms.

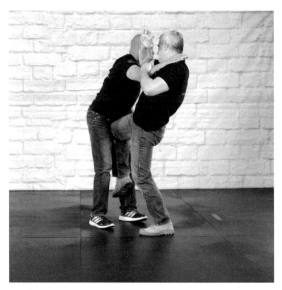

Straight-knee counterattack against a rear naked choke attempt.

Immediately deliver a knee from your rear leg to the attacker's exposed groin or midsection, followed by additional retzev counterattacks.

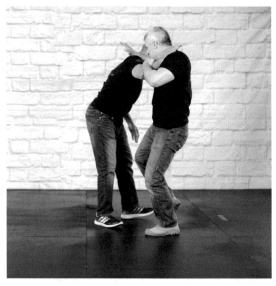

Straight-knee counterattack followed by an outside chop against a rear naked choke attempt.

Follow the initial debilitating straight-knee counterattack with an outside chop, along with additional retzev counterattacks, if needed.

Professional Rear Naked Choke on the Ground

Surviving on the ground sometimes means choking an opponent. The professional rear naked choke serves this purpose well. Keep in mind that any ground combatives that require you to lock up with an opponent will place you in jeopardy of a third party attacking you, especially with stomps to the head.

When there is no choice but to go to the ground, "taking" the adversary's back—placing your chest to his back with his torso between your legs—is the most advantageous position, provided you are not facing multiple opponents. The advantage of this position is that you have an array of combative strikes at your disposal to facilitate a choke, including elbows and forearm strikes to the back of the neck, eye gouges, and heel kicks to your adversary's groin and abdomen.

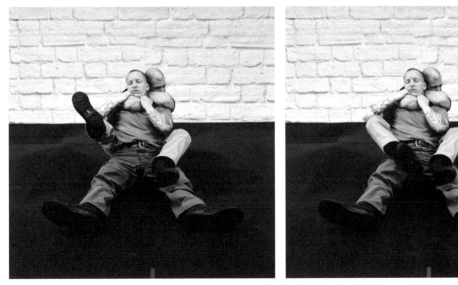

Professional rear naked choke on the ground with facilitating heel kicks to debilitate the opponent.

Combative Counters to Defensive Measures against Your Rear Naked Choke Attempt

If the adversary defends your attempted rear naked choke by yanking down on your choking arm, you may use your other arm to insert and apply the choke. Alternatively, if the adversary is resisting your choke, rake his eyes with your nonchoking arm to expose his throat and neck. Then you can apply a forearm choke, crook-of-the-elbow choke, or professional rear naked choke. You may administer horizontal elbow strikes and forearm strikes to the base or back of the adversary's skull to disorient him, facilitating your choke options. Note: You may also grab your own clothing, reinforcing your hold on him while repositioning your other arm underneath his chin to execute an opposite-arm choke. Basically, this is switching one choking arm for the other.

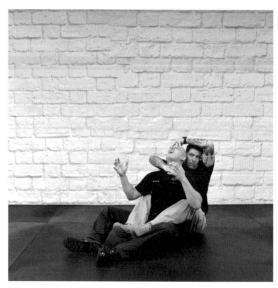

Professional rear naked choke on the ground preceded by eye-rake facilitator.

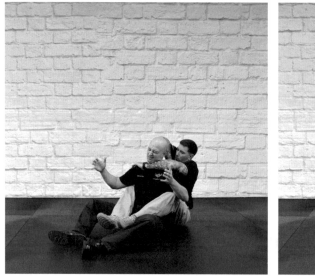
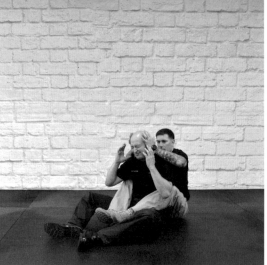

Rear naked professional choke on the ground. Facilitators also include palm-heel strikes to ears or horizontal elbow strikes to head.

Standing Professional Underneath Choke

The standing professional underneath choke may be used if you succeed in getting the opponent's level down by kneeing him in the midsection, thigh, or groin—or by otherwise staggering him. It is important to debilitate the opponent to prevent him from defending the choke. The best way to do this is to strike his groin. Then, to apply the choke, knife your arm underneath the opponent's throat to catch his neck in the crook of your elbow. Immediately begin to squeeze his neck between your forearm and biceps. As you cinch the choke, wrap your other arm around the back of his head to complete a figure-4 "vise grip" similar to the professional rear naked choke you mastered in the previous tactics.

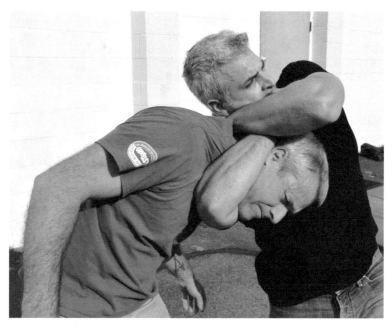

Standing professional underneath choke.

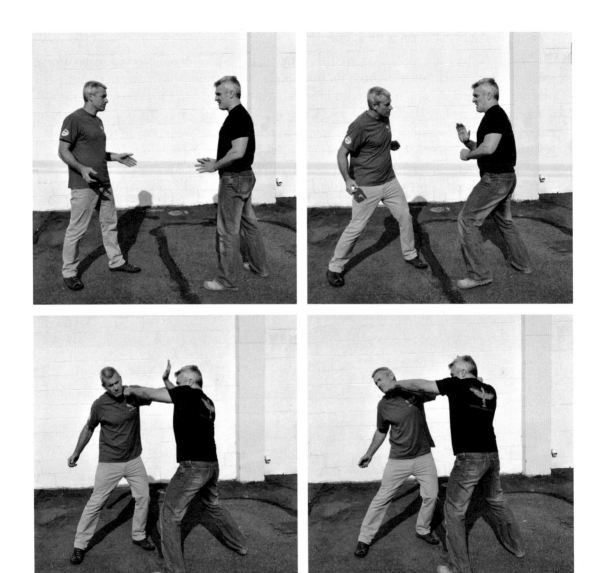

Standing professional underneath choke used in defending a hook punch.

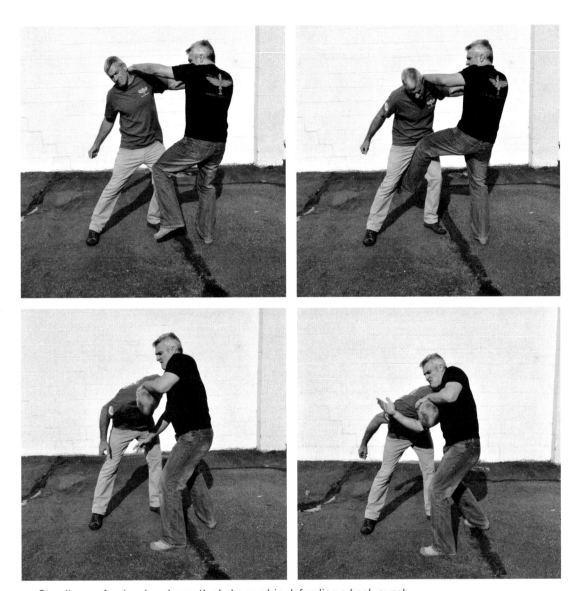

Standing professional underneath choke used in defending a hook punch.

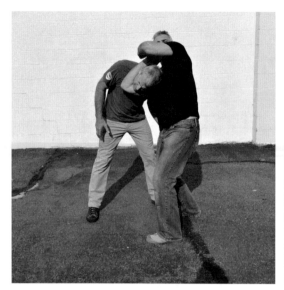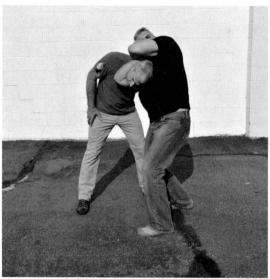

Standing professional underneath choke used in defending a hook punch.

Standing Triangle Choke (Kata Gatame)

The standing triangle choke, or *kata gatame*, is a variation of the previously depicted crook-of-the-elbow choke and professional rear naked choke. Which of these variations you decide to use will likely depend on your arm length. The tactic depicted is orchestrated out of a straight sliding parry punch defense.

Example: Sliding Parry While Stepping "Off the Line" into Modified Standing Triangle Choke

This defense allows you to deflect an incoming rear punch or cross while simultaneously moving slightly away from the punch. At the same time, deliver your own counterattack strike to the throat, chin, nose, midsection, or groin. Note that this defense and the following related triangle defenses enable a defender to use the same defense (albeit with opposite movements) against a straight punch to close on the assailant and neutralize the threat. Your hand leads your body defense to redirect the adversary's punch by sliding down your adversary's right arm, while your right arm delivers a half-roundhouse counterpunch to the throat, chin, or nose.

To defend a straight punch from your left outlet stance, step to your left while bringing your left cupped hand diagonally across your face close to your right shoulder. The key is to deflect and step off the line, moving both feet together, while simultaneously counterpunching. Do not lunge; keep your feet equidistant by moving them the same distance. You may also punch low to the assailant's body, targeting his liver, or deliver a hand strike to his groin. (These last two counterstrikes are useful if an assailant has a height advantage and you cannot readily reach his head to counterattack.) This defense is followed up with trapping the adversary's right arm and placing him in a standing triangle "blood choke." Be sure to secure his right shoulder tightly against his right carotid artery while using the radial bone of your right arm against his left carotid artery. As depicted in the photos, bury your head behind your opponent's head to add pressure and protect your face.

Slip your counterpunch arm around the assailant's neck, placing your biceps against one of the main arteries (the common right and left carotids) carrying blood to the brain through the carotid sheath, while trapping the assailant's shoulder against the other main artery and clamping down in a figure-4 to execute a blood choke. Last, several strong takedowns are available from this triangular choke position, including taking the assailant down into formidable choke positions on the ground. In addition, there are a number of devastating throws one may use to break the assailant from the modified triangle hold. Note: For the sliding parry defense, if you misread the assailant's straight punch—for instance, he throws a left punch instead of a right—stepping off the line properly will still allow the defense to work. You will have avoided the punch with a body defense (stepping off the line of attack) while counterattacking. In essence, you will "split" the assailant's hands with your counterpunch. The immediate danger is that you are still to your adversary's liveside: he still may have the ability to mount an effective counterattack. The preferred defense is always to move to his deadside, minimizing his ability to counterattack.

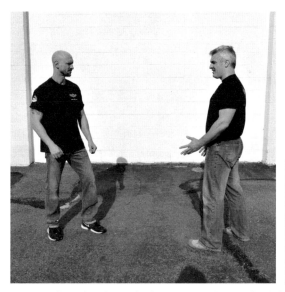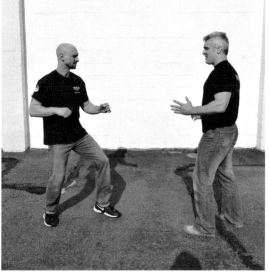

Standing triangle choke (kata gatame) used in defending a straight punch.

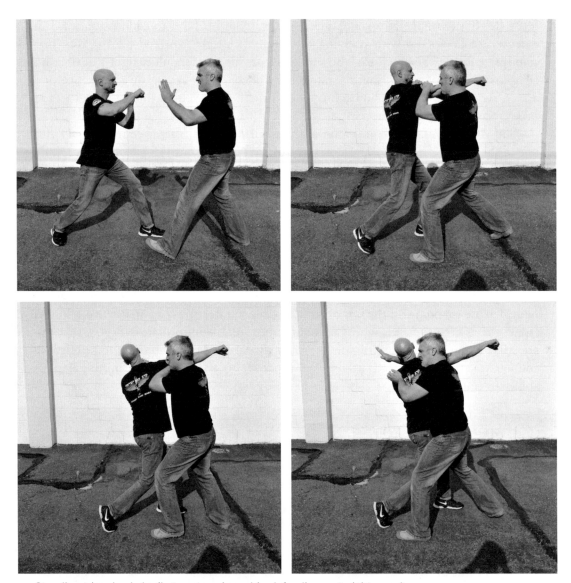

Standing triangle choke (kata gatame) used in defending a straight punch.

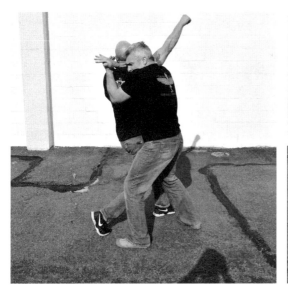 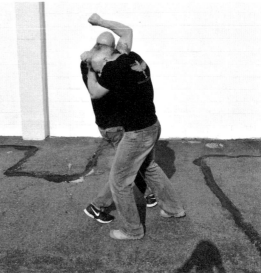

Standing triangle choke (kata gatame) used in defending a straight punch.

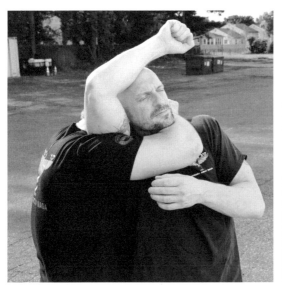 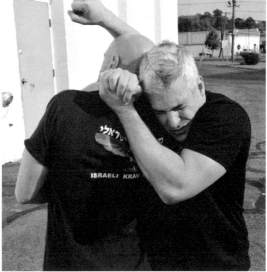

Standing triangle choke (kata gatame), close-up.

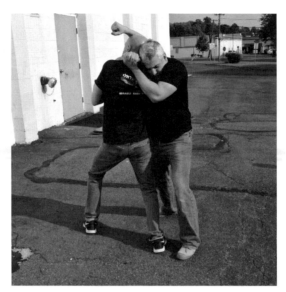

Standing triangle choke (kata gatame), alternative view.

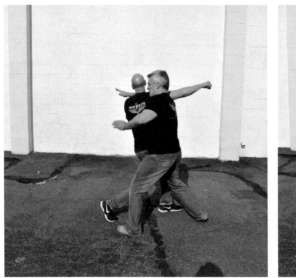
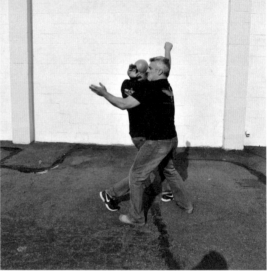

Standing triangle choke (kata gatame), professional rear naked choke-hold grip variation.

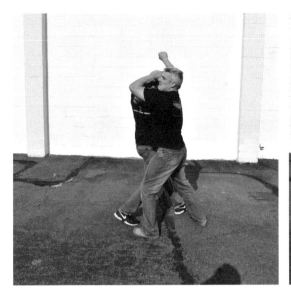
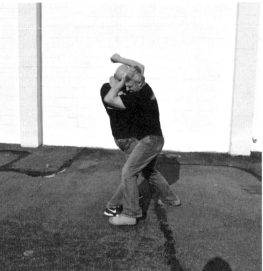
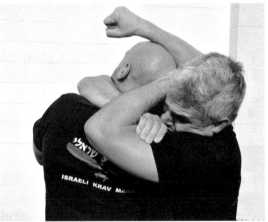

Standing triangle choke (kata gatame), professional rear naked choke-hold grip variation.

Ground Triangle Choke (Kata Gatame Variation)

The ground triangle choke, or *kata gatame*, is similar to your standing triangle choke tactic; however, it is even more powerful because you can use your body weight and gravity to aid you in the choke. The key is to secure the choke and immediately drive your shoulder through the opponent's shoulder and biceps to apply pressure on his near-side carotid. At the same time, use the blade of your arm to apply pressure to his other carotid. Create a strong base with your legs by spreading them apart and pushing forward on the balls of your feet. You may further cinch the choke by spinning your lower body (in this case clockwise to tighten a right-arm choke). If you feel balanced, once you cinch the choke after you have moved your feet to an optimum choke angle, you may cross one foot over the other. This gives you a narrow base to add concentrated body-weight pressure in the choke to further drive your shoulder into the opponent and optimize the choke.

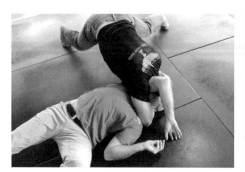 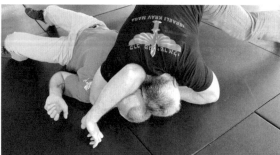

Ground triangle choke (kata gatame) variation.

Collar Chokes

Krav maga has ten collar chokes tied into the curriculum. As you will recall, krav maga's military origins take into account a military tunic, blouse, or sling that could be readily available to apply a choke in a hand-to-hand combat situation. Presented are two of the easiest collar chokes to master and apply.

Cross-Collar Choke

The cross-collar choke is extremely effective and adds insult to injury. In the photo series, the defender preempts a hook punch by delivering an inverted straight punch to the attacker's head to momentarily stun him, setting up a cross-collar choke.

Your right fist punches into the opponent's jaw or carotid. Your hand is close to the attacker's collar, hence the opportunity to deliver a cross-collar choke. Seize the left collar with your right hand and the right collar with your left hand. Once you have secured the collar on both sides, punch across the neckline with your right hand and into the lower portion of the neck with your left hand (below your right hand) in an X pattern, to apply extreme pressure against both sides of the neck. This will cut blood flow through the carotid arteries to effectuate the blood choke.

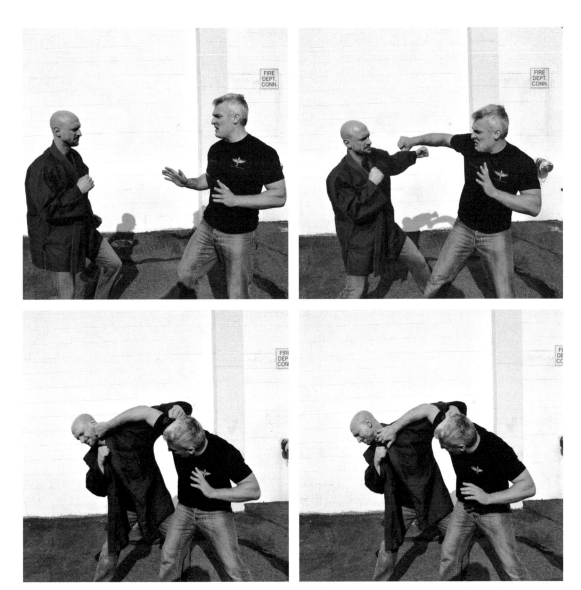

Cross-collar choke used in defending a hook punch. Note: You must choke him efficiently and quickly to prevent his counterattack to your eyes.

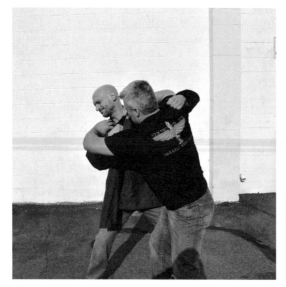
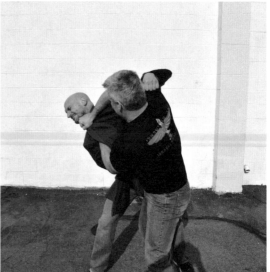

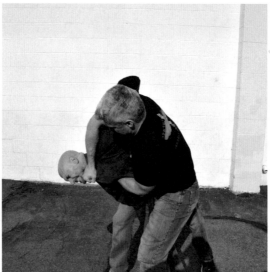

Cross-collar choke used in defending a hook punch. Note: You must choke him efficiently and quickly to prevent his counterattack to your eyes.

Knuckles Choke

Similar to the cross-collar choke, the knuckles choke applies pressure on both sides of the neck against the carotid sheath. You can seize the opportunity by kneeing the opponent in the groin to gain an entry. You must reach deep into the opponent's collar, grasping the collar to enable a strong grip and correct positioning of your knuckles.

Once you secure the collar, raise your arms slightly and sharply dig your knuckles into the opponent's carotid as you rotate your hands inward. Beware of the opponent's possible defenses and counterattacks. In other words, think how you might defend this tactic as a kravist—as you should for all krav maga tactics in this book.

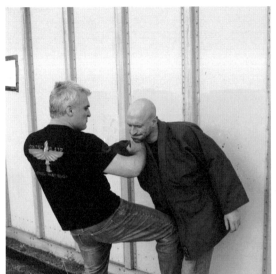 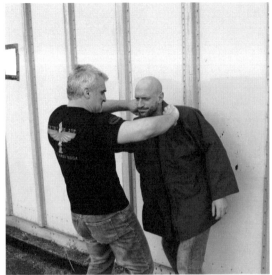

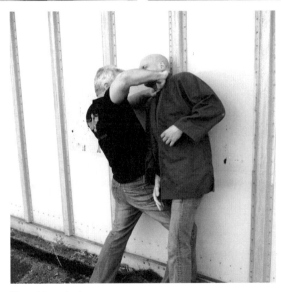

Knuckles choke.

Chapter 4

Lower-Body Combatives

Combative Family #8: Straight Kicks and Knees

Your lower body houses the most powerful fighting weapons you can use at maximum fighting range. Your knees, shinbones, and the balls of your feet (especially when clad in shoes) serve as hard and durable striking surfaces. When you kick or knee your opponent, you use your body's largest muscle groups, including the gluteals, quadriceps, and hamstrings. The leg is usually two times the mass of the arm—if not more—hence the added power. If, as with punching, you put your entire body mass and strength behind your kick or knee, you can deliver a devastating blow, no matter your size or weight.

If I face an unavoidable physical confrontation, provided I have the proper range and timing, I am going to preemptively kick the assailant. My preference is a side kick targeting the aggressor's knee or a straight kick to his lead knee or groin. I will follow this combative with whatever additional retzev combatives are necessary to stop the threat. By using a linear preemptive kick, I limit the defensive reactions I must consider. In other words, it doesn't matter what type of combative the assailant throws at me. I target his vulnerable anatomy with my longest-range intercept weapon: a kick. In addition, most street thugs do not train to defend against a quick, powerful low-line kick. By moving toward me, the aggressor is placing his weight on his lead leg. Kicking the knee of a weight-bearing leg is devastating and one of the best methods to stop an attack.

You can perform krav maga kicks low, at the torso, and at the head. To deliver head kicks, you'll need flexibility, balance, and enough strength to lift your leg. The Israel Defense Force, in developing its krav maga program, set up tested candidates, many of whom were talented martial artists, to run extensive distances with full combat loads. After an exhausting run in combat gear, the candidates were told to defend against an attack using whatever techniques they felt most comfortable. Few test candidates favoring high kicks could perform them. Their physical exhaustion prior to the fighting tests made high kicking extremely difficult.

The IDF recognized the need to use fighting techniques that would work for all trainees, especially under trying circumstances. Therefore, low kicks combined with upper body combatives became integral to krav maga training. When asked if krav maga favored kicks to the head, Imi replied, "Of course we kick to the head, but first we beat him to the ground, and then we kick to the head."

For most kicks, you'll make contact using the ball of your foot or your heel. To practice and prepare your feet for striking, curl your toes up toward you, exposing the heel, and repeatedly pound the ground with the ball of your foot. Note this heel exercise is a combative kick in itself, the stomp.

For all straight kicks and knees, think of your kneecap as a direction finder or pointer. Wherever the knee is pointed, the kick or knee will follow. Hip alignment is paramount to keeping your leg on target. Note: Do not fully extend the kicking leg unless you are impacting a target. Rather, only extend about 90 percent. As with punches, you can hyperextend your knee by locking the joint.

Lead Straight Offensive Kick

To practice the lead straight offensive kick, starting from your left outlet stance, take the longest possible step forward with your left leg. As you step, turn your right foot out approximately 90 degrees. Note that your left outlet stance facilitates the movement of your base-leg foot. Notice how your body elongates and your nonkicking leg naturally pivots out with your toes pointed to your right. (Although the optimal turn is 90 degrees, some people experience knee discomfort when they turn the knee this far.) Turning out on the ball of the foot of your rear base leg will thrust your hips forward, giving you maximum extension and power using glicha, or a sliding step, to carry your body weight through the kick. This enables you to throw your body mass behind the kick. You will actually launch the kick from low to high or "under the radar screen" of your opponent's vision. Connect with the ball of your left foot against your target. Do not raise your knee up and then push out to kick. Let your body move your lead leg in a natural upward trajectory. Do not snap or thrust the kick toward the target. After impact, land with your kicking leg forward. If you are in a de-escalation or passive stance, as you launch the kick, thrust your hands forward and up into a fighting position, as this accelerates your entire body through the kick. When defending, try to keep your hands up the entire time. Many people unconsciously drop their hands to improve their balance. (Note: You can practice keeping your hands up by grabbing your shirt collar as you kick.)

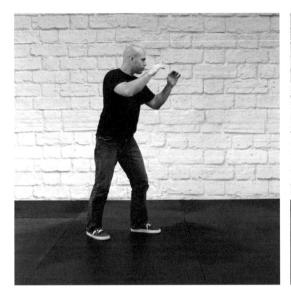
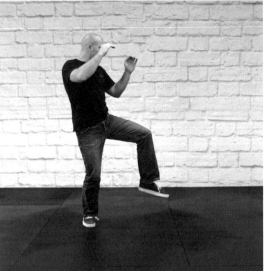
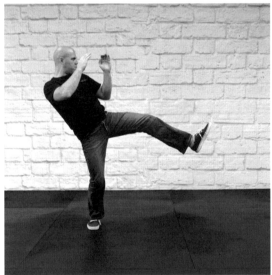

Lead straight offensive kick. Note the base-leg turn.

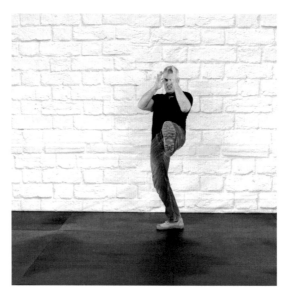

Lead straight offensive kick, front view. Note the base-leg turn.

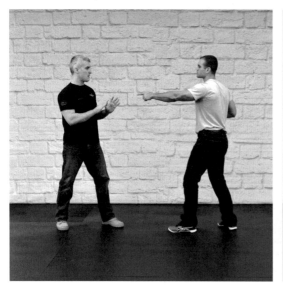 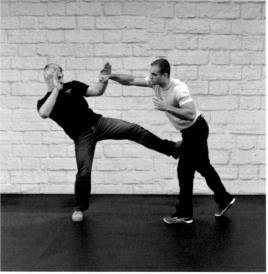

Lead straight offensive kick used in defending a straight punch. Note the base-leg turn.

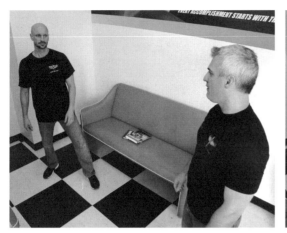 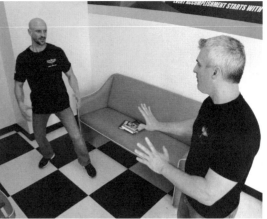

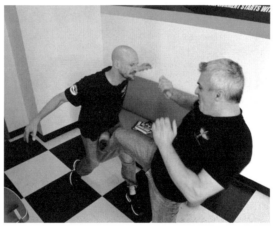

Lead straight offensive kick used preemptively in defending an encroaching threat.

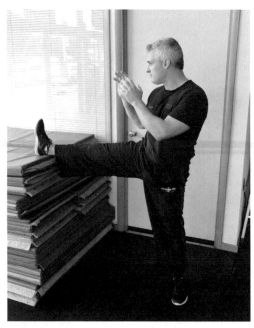

Straight-kick stretch.

Rear Straight Kick

For the rear straight kick, you'll use kicking and base-leg movements similar to the ones you used for the lead straight kick. These will maximize your reach and kicking power. As you close the distance to your opponent following your kick, linear straight punches and palm-heel strikes are strong follow-up combatives into elbow and knee strikes to facilitate retzev. In practice, from your left outlet stance, take the largest step you can with your right leg and remain in that position. You will notice how your body elongates again and your nonkicking base leg pivots to approximately a 90-degree angle, with your toes pointed to your right. To actually perform the kick, thrust your rear leg out as though you are pushing the ball of your foot through a target, again, "under the radar screen." Let your body move your rear leg in a natural upward trajectory. Do not snap or thrust the kick toward the target. After impact, land with your kicking leg forward. If you are in a de-escalation or passive stance, as you launch the kick, thrust your hands forward and up into a fighting position, as this accelerates your entire body through the kick. When defending, as always, try to keep your hands up the entire time. Many people unconsciously drop their hands to improve their balance. As you kick, keep your hands up to protect your head. To enhance your footwork and balance, learn to deliver the kick and then retreat into an opposite fighting stance. As your kicking leg touches the ground, use the retreating footwork you learned with your straight punches to move your body backward.

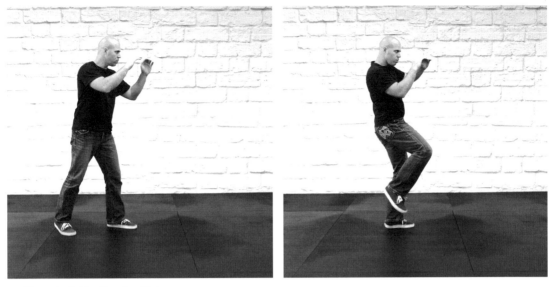

Rear straight offensive kick.

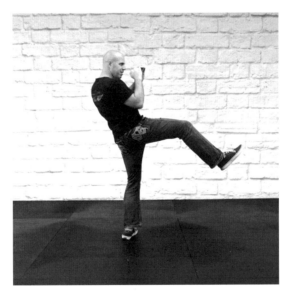

Rear straight offensive kick. Note the base-leg turn.

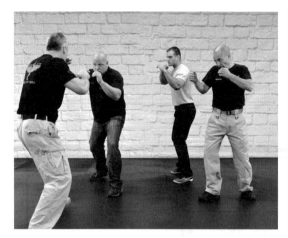 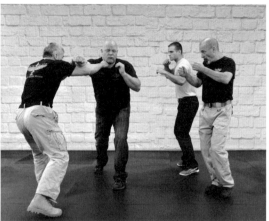

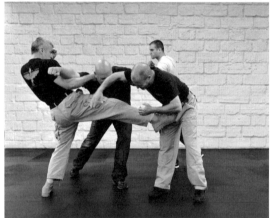

Rear straight offensive kick used when defending against multiple opponents. Note the base-leg turn.

Using Pocket Change as a Distraction, Combined with a Rear Straight Kick

To ambush your opponent with a rear straight kick, you may launch pocket change or any other distraction, including liquid from a cup, spittle, and chewing gum, at his face. It is best to keep the distraction hidden and not telegraph your intent. Conceal the loose change in your hand slightly behind your back or at your side. Do not make it obvious that you have something in your hand. You may launch the change using an underhand throw (which I prefer) or palm-down throw. As you launch the change, begin your kicking motion using a sliding step with your base leg, propelling your entire kick through the opponent. Target his groin or his midsection. Be sure to properly align your leg to kick and use the ball of your foot to make impact. Follow up with retzev combatives as necessary.

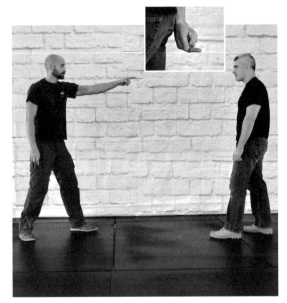
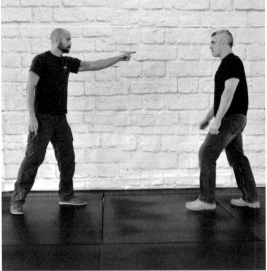

Rear straight offensive kick combined with using pocket change as a distraction.

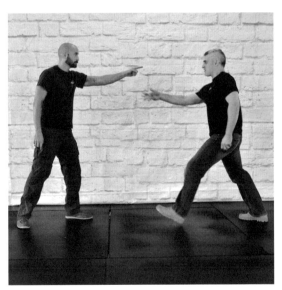
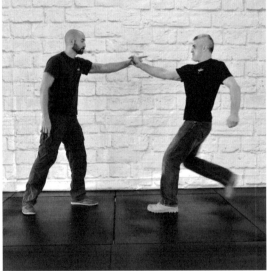

Rear straight offensive kick combined with using pocket change as a distraction.

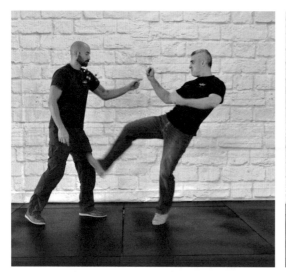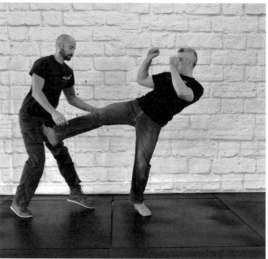

Rear straight offensive kick combined with using pocket change as a distraction. Note the base-leg turn.

Straight Shin Kick

The straight shin kick may also be delivered making contact to the opponent's groin with your shin. The kick mechanics remain the same: turn the base-leg for maximum extension and weight transfer through the kick. If you direct your leg between your opponent's legs and kick upward, your leg will naturally trace the inside of the opponent's thigh to impact his groin.

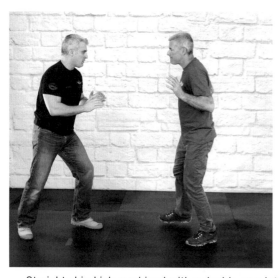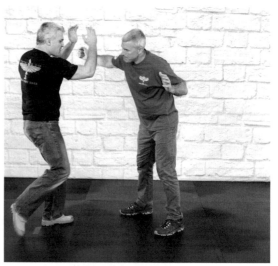

Straight shin kick combined with a double-arm interception in defending a hook punch.

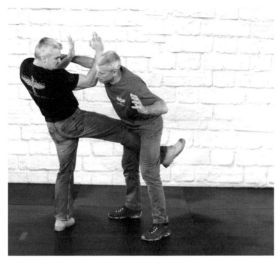

Straight shin kick combined with a double-arm interception in defending a hook punch. Note the base-leg turn.

Lead Straight Offensive Kick with Glicha Shuffle Step

The lead straight kick may be enhanced by using a shuffle step. Essentially, you are replacing your lead foot position with your rear foot position. This movement optimally drives your entire body weight through the attacker. In other words, your rear foot is shuffling forward or "kicking out" your lead foot, which then delivers the strike. This shuffle step sends your entire mass in motion, launching through the opponent with the ball of your foot.

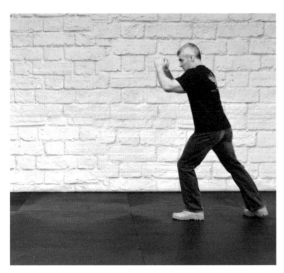
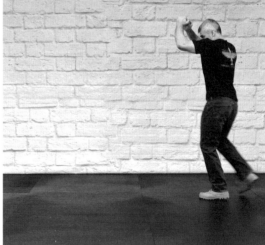

Lead straight offensive kick with glicha shuffle step.

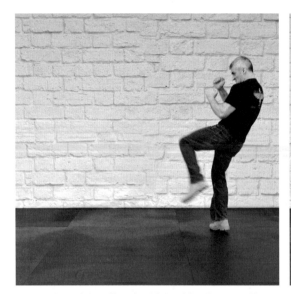 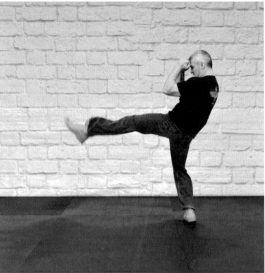

Lead straight offensive kick with glicha shuffle step. Note the base-leg turn.

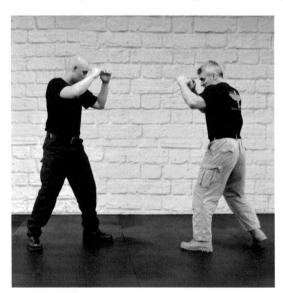 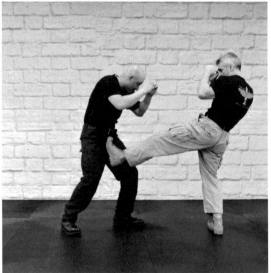

Lead straight offensive kick with glicha shuffle step. Preemptory kick. Note the base-leg turn.

Rear Straight Offensive Kick with Secoul Sliding Step

The rear straight kick with secoul places your entire body in motion to maximize your reach, momentum, and kinetic energy. This is achieved by using a sliding step with your lead base leg. Essentially, you are stepping forward while simultaneously pivoting on your lead base leg. The kick is a slide (secoul), not a jump. By sliding on the lead base-leg pivot foot, you are positioned to optimally drive your entire body weight through the attacker. In other words, your entire mass is in motion, launching through the opponent with the ball of your foot.

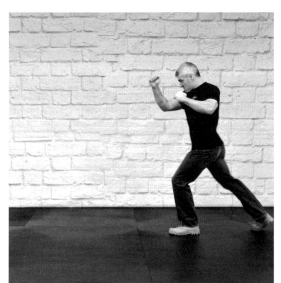 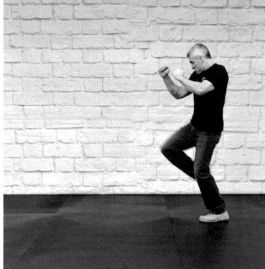

Rear straight offensive kick with secoul sliding step.

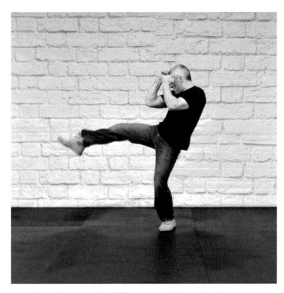

Rear straight offensive kick with secoul sliding step. Note the base-leg turn.

Straight Scissors Kick

The straight scissors kick is an advanced kick using your kicking leg to both spring you into the air and deliver the kick. This kick is most often used in combination with the cavalier #1 takedown. As you jump upward with your kicking leg, your other leg should also rise up, or "jackknife," to provide more lift. Make contact with the ball of your kicking foot or the shin of your kicking leg, depending on the distance.

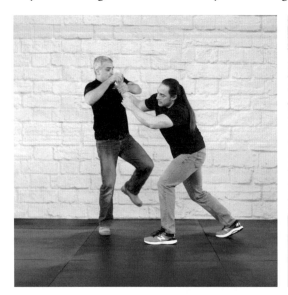 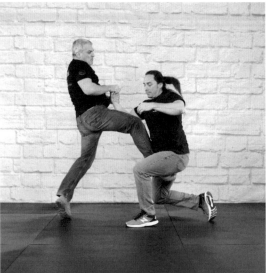

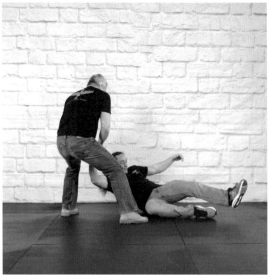

Straight scissors kick.

Retreating Straight Kick

The retreating straight kick may be used when you attempt to de-escalate a situation by moving away from the conflict, and yet the opponent follows you. Step back with your lead leg. As you step back, you will switch lead legs. Open up your hip by placing the foot of your rear leg at a 90-degree angle. This is the pivotal (pun intended) base-leg turn for maximum reach and power.

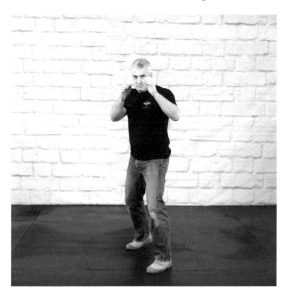 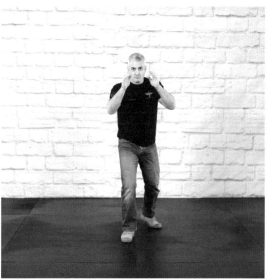

Retreating straight kick.

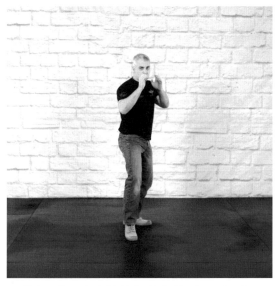 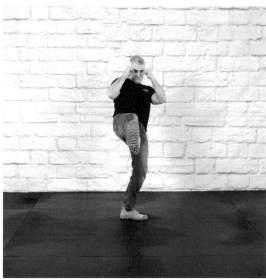

Retreating straight kick. Note the base-leg turn.

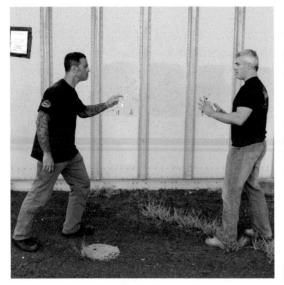 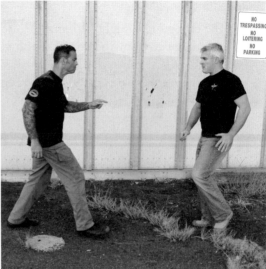

Retreating straight kick against an encroaching threat.

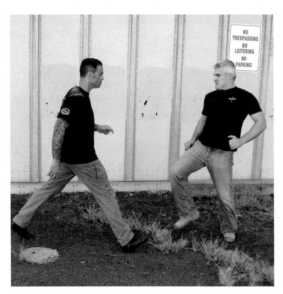 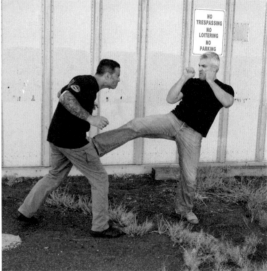

Retreating straight kick against an encroaching threat. Note the base-leg turn.

Straight Knee

Once you know how to deliver straight kicks, you know how to deliver a straight knee. Knee attacks provide some of the most punishing strikes and a strong finish to any technique. Shorter-range elbow strikes work extremely well when combined with knee strikes and are strong follow-up combatives into retzev. Knee your opponent with the same technique you use to kick. Rather than make contact with your foot, however, you'll jam your kneecap into your target. By returning to your left outlet stance, you will rechamber your knee to provide additional powerful and debilitating strikes.

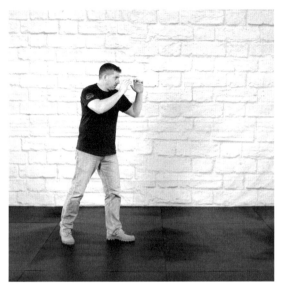 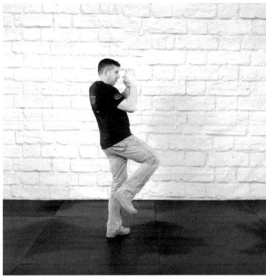

Rear straight knee.

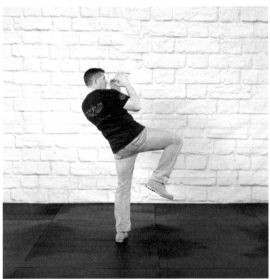 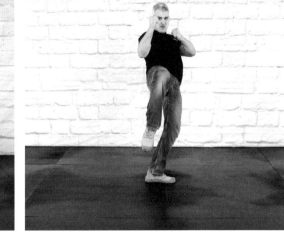

Rear straight knee. Note the base-leg turn.

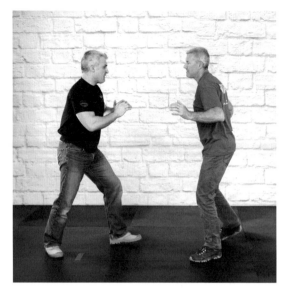
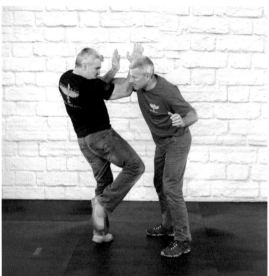
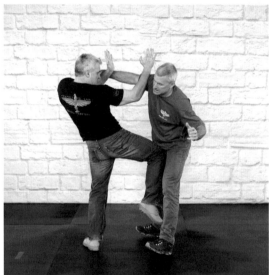

Rear straight knee combined with a double-arm interception in defending a hook punch. Note the base-leg turn.

Combined Trap and Rear Straight Knee against Attacker Standing in Left Outlet Stance

This combined offensive knee and trap combative is designed to catch and control your opponent's arms while delivering a devastating lead knee to the opponent's groin, thigh, or midsection, followed by additional retzev combatives. If your opponent has his arms close together, executing a trap by grabbing and pulling his arms to you can be highly effective. Grab both his wrists and yank him into you as you propel a straight knee strike into his midsection with a proper 90-degree turn of the base leg.

While not depicted, if your opponent has his hands wide apart, you can split his hands by putting your palms together and stabbing your arms between his arms, driving them farther apart as you deliver a straight knee with the proper base-leg turn.

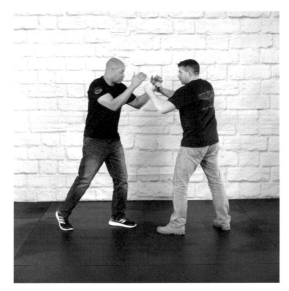 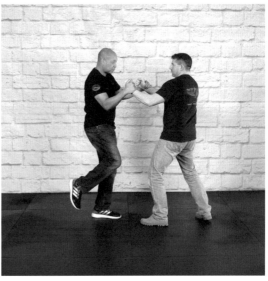

Combined trap and rear straight knee against a standing attacker.

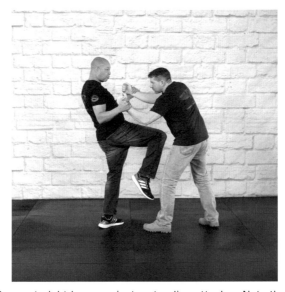

Combined trap and rear straight knee against a standing attacker. Note the base-leg turn.

Rear Knee Combined with an Uppercut Punch against a Takedown

This combined offensive knee and uppercut combative is designed to defeat a tackle takedown attempt. Using correct timing as the attacker lowers his level and closes on you, deliver a devastating straight knee strike to his head. The knee is naturally followed up by an uppercut punch simultaneously as your lead leg touches down to the ground. Note: You could substitute the uppercut punch with an inside chop.

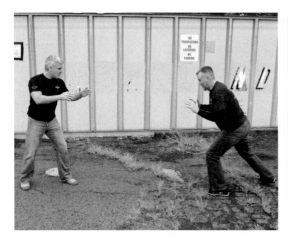 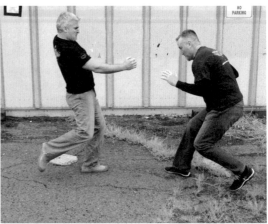

Rear straight knee combined with an uppercut punch against a takedown.

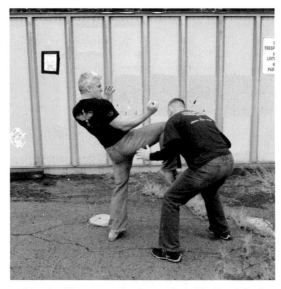

Rear straight knee combined with an uppercut punch against a takedown. Note the base-leg turn.

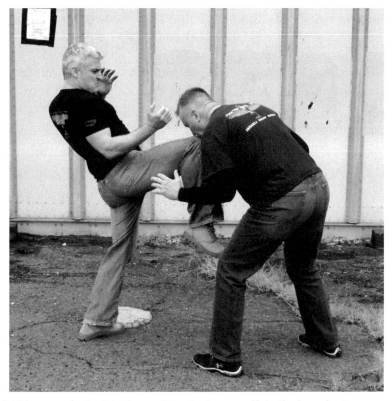

Rear straight knee against a takedown attempt, close-up. Note the base-leg turn.

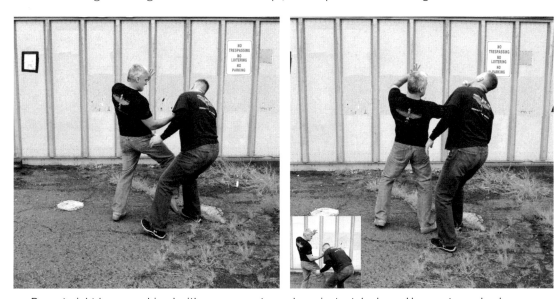

Rear straight knee combined with an uppercut punch against a takedown. Uppercut punch, close-up. Note the base-leg turn.

Combative Family #9: Stomps, Side Kicks, Rear Defensive Kicks, and Linear Ground Kicks

Using your heel to kick someone is likely your most powerful combative. You can recruit all the muscles of your leg while simultaneously moving your body weight through the kick. The following kick options harness this instinctive mechanism.

Heel Stomp

If you knock the attacker to the ground while you are still standing, the heel stomp is a simple and highly effective combative targeting the top of the attacker's foot or other exposed areas such as the groin, head, and throat (in a deadly force encounter), as well as the ribs, kidneys, or hands. Note: You can also strike his Achilles if he is kneeling, which will likely hobble him.

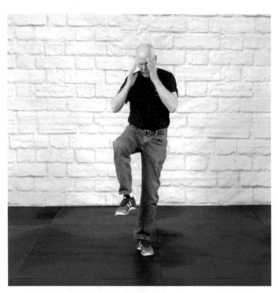 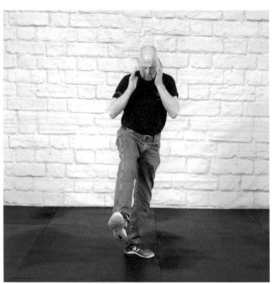

Heel stomp.

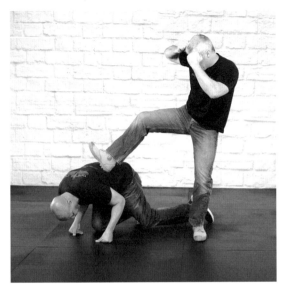 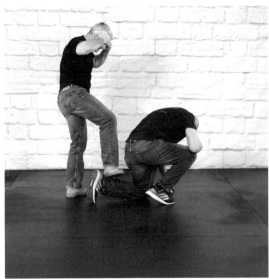

Heel stomp targeting vulnerable anatomy.

Side Kick

The side kick may be the most important krav maga tool in your arsenal, provided you are at the correct range to use it. The side kick and rear straight defensive kick build your arsenal of combatives, enabling you to kick a threat to your side or rear. The side kick and rear defensive kicks will become some of your most formidable striking weapons. The side kick is highly effective against lateral attacks such as straight punches, where you can use the kick's superior reach and power against the attacker's lead knee, thighs, or midsection. If you vary your outlet stance or "cheat" by positioning your feet almost perpendicular to your opponent, the side kick can target an opponent in front of you. Execute the side kick with your lead leg, which is closer to your target. Once again, pivoting and aligning the base leg in the appropriate direction are essential to maximize reach and power. To perform the side kick, raise your lead kicking leg until it is bent 90 degrees and your thigh is parallel to the ground. Deliver the kick by thrusting your raised leg out, pointing the heel toward the target and curling the toes toward your body. Keep your foot parallel with the ground as you make contact. As with every other kick, your body weight must shift forward into your target by sliding on the ball of the foot of your baseleg.

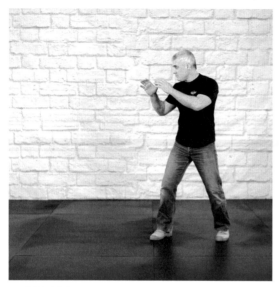 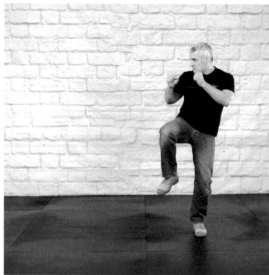

Side kick.

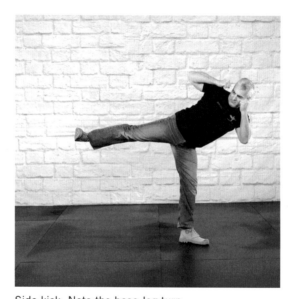

Side kick. Note the base-leg turn.

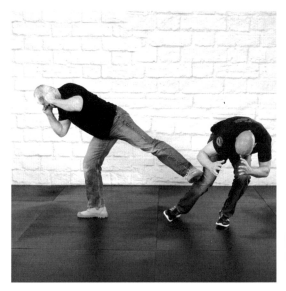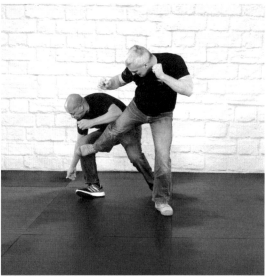

Side kick targeting the knee. Note the base-leg turn.

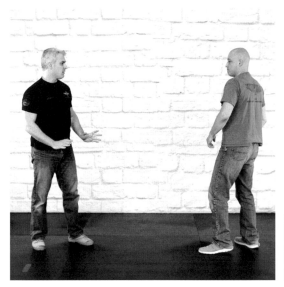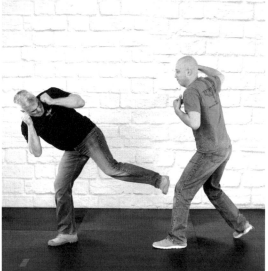

Side kick targeting the knee to preempt an attack. Note the base-leg turn.

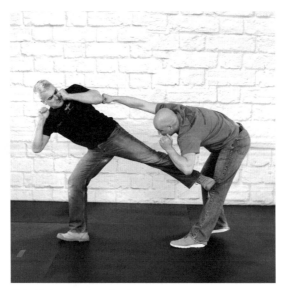

Side kick targeting the knee to preempt an attack.
Note the base-leg turn.

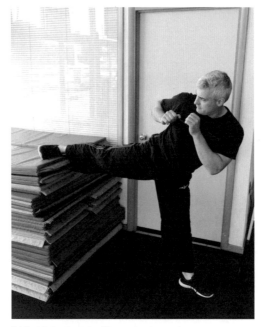

Side kick stretch. Note the base-leg turn.

Rear Defensive Kick

Targets for the rear defensive kick include the knees, thighs, groin, midsection, and solar plexus. Higher kicks can target the neck and head. To recognize a threat from behind, turn your head in the direction of your attacker. Even though your upper torso will naturally lean away from the kick, drive your body through the target by sliding toward the target on the foot of your base leg. Thrust your foot into your opponent, connecting with your heel, as you did with the side kick. You may connect with your foot parallel to the ground or with your toes pointed to the ground.

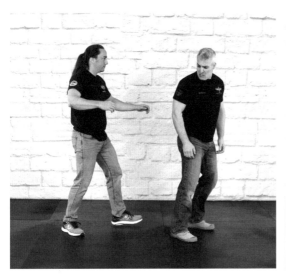
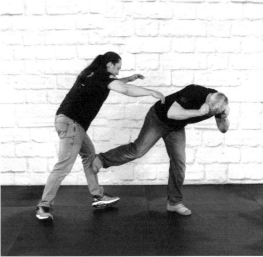

Rear defensive kick used in defending an attempted grab or choke from behind.

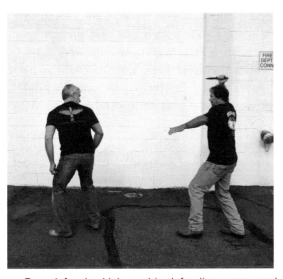
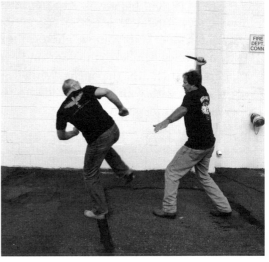

Rear defensive kick used in defending a rear overhead edged-weapon attack.

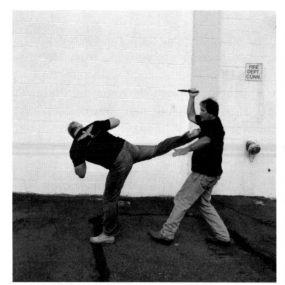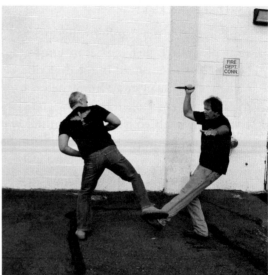

Rear defensive kick used in defending a rear overhead edged-weapon attack.

Stepping Side Kick

The stepping side kick is an extremely powerful combative that enables you to kick an opponent who is to your side, while covering a longer distance. Targets include the shin, knee, thigh, midsection, or head. The stepping side kick is an effective combative for striking an opponent at a greater distance using a step (secoul) by varying your left outlet stance. You can also "cheat" by positioning your feet almost perpendicular to your opponent, rather than retain the left outlet stance, where your feet are positioned about 45 degrees to your opponent. Execute the stepping side kick with the lead leg, closest to your target. Your rear leg or base leg crosses behind your lead leg as you prepare to launch the kick. Shift your weight to your rear leg, angle your heel toward the opponent, extend your leg parallel to the floor, and make contact with the heel. The heel of the step-ping leg must face the opponent. While you may lean back slightly because your kicking leg is raised with your thigh parallel to the ground, make sure your weight is coming forward and through your target.

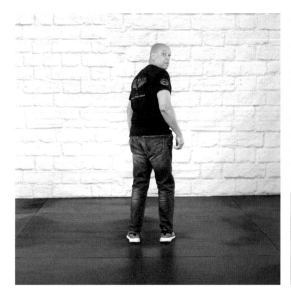
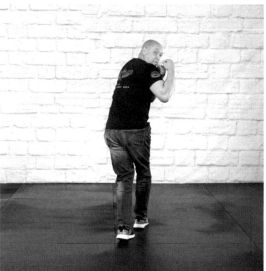

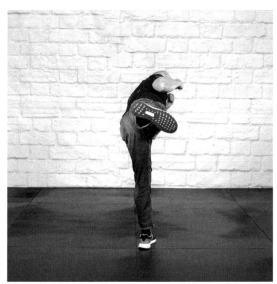

Stepping side kick.

Straight Heel Kick from the Ground

Even when you're on the ground, you can successfully launch a lead straight heel kick against a standing opponent. As soon as you fall to the ground, protect your head, using arm positioning similar to that of your outlet stance. Although you may periodically drop your arms to the ground to move your body back away from your opponent or rotate your body to meet a threat from a different angle, keep your arms in position to protect your head as often as you can. As you kick, keep your base leg against the ground for leverage. Thrust the kick out with your kicking leg. Use your upper back and shoulders as a launching platform, allowing your torso to lift off the ground and put its weight behind the kick. Make contact with either the heel or ball of your foot, and recoil quickly so your opponent cannot catch your leg. Launching this kick from the ground becomes an offensive movement due to your angle of attack against a standing opponent.

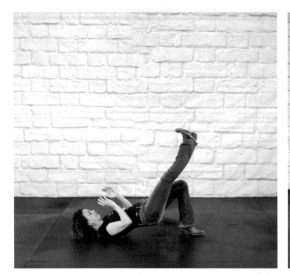
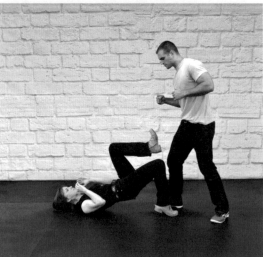

Straight heel kick from the ground.

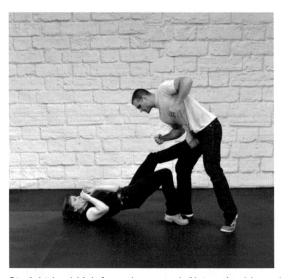

Straight heel kick from the ground. Note raised base-leg heel.

Ground Side Kick

The ground side kick works well if you find yourself on the ground with your attacker standing over you. The attacker's knees, thighs, and groin usually present the best targets when in this position. If opportune, you can also increase the effectiveness of this combative by hooking the attacker's heel with your lower leg to immobilize the knee just prior to impact, thereby increasing trauma to the knee. To execute the ground side kick, keep both hands raised in a defensive posture and one leg on the ground. Kick sideways in an upward motion, curling your toes toward you and connecting with your heel. You may wish to place one forearm on the ground to establish a strong kicking base with good balance. Keep your nonkicking leg flush against the ground prior to the kick. As you kick, this base leg (with your foot on the ground) may rise slightly off the ground to give you leverage. Remember: lift your foot upward to make contact with the targeted area.

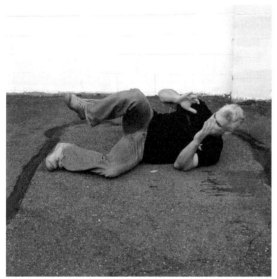 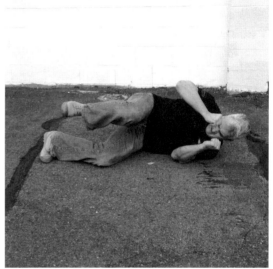

Ground side kick.

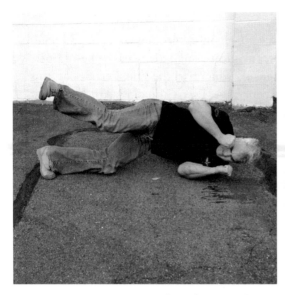 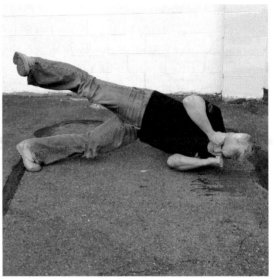

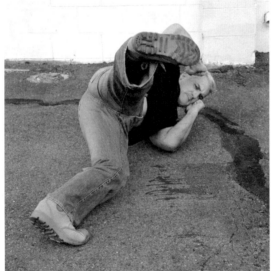

Ground side kick. Note body raise for maximum reach and power.

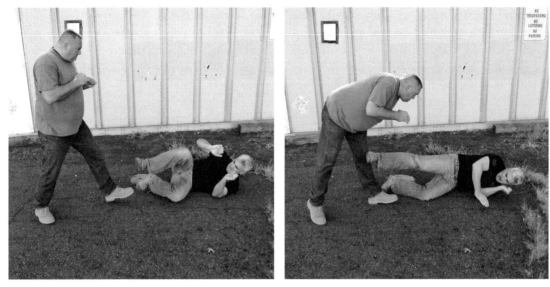

Ground side kick rising on shoulder. Note body raise for maximum reach and power.

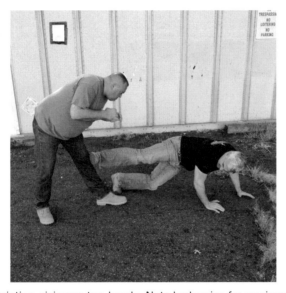

Ground side kick variation, rising on two hands. Note body raise for maximum reach and power.

Standing Straight Instep Kick

The straight instep kick is highly effective against a standing opponent's knee when you are upright or on the ground, either on your back or on your side. The kick is delivered using your instep against the attacker's leg, preferably his knee. Your kicking foot is therefore parallel to the ground with your instep facing skyward. The standing straight instep kick may be delivered anytime you are positioned to your opponent's rear. Target the side of his knee for maximum damage or, if the angle dictates, the crook of his knee to buckle his knee inward. This kick forces the opponent forward to the ground, exposing him to other combatives, should they be necessary.

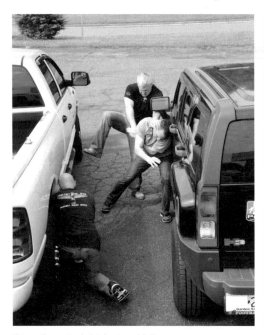 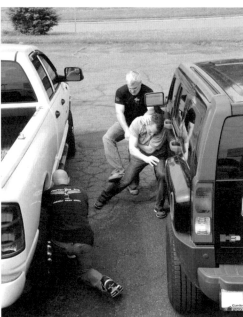

Standing straight instep kick.

Straight Instep Kick from the Ground

To launch the straight instep kick when on your side, use your lower leg or the leg closer to the ground. To optimize the kick, try to "bridge" with your body, rising up on your base leg and opposite shoulder to lift your body off the ground and drive through the opponent.

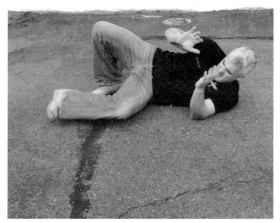 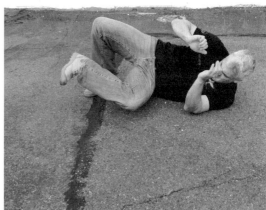

Straight instep kick from the ground.

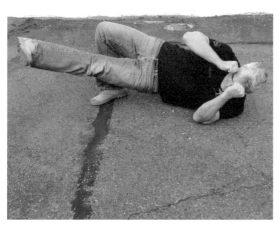 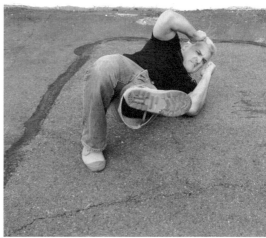

Straight instep kick from the ground. Note body raise for maximum reach and power.

Combatives Family #10: Roundhouse Kicks, Sweeps, Inside Slap Kicks, and Roundhouse Ground Kicks

Roundhouse lower body combatives are highly effective strikes targeting an opponent's Achilles tendon, knee, thigh, groin, ribs, liver, kidneys, and head. In the late 1980s, Grandmaster Gidon introduced kicks utilizing the shin in addition to continuing kicks with the ball of the foot.

Lead Roundhouse Kick

The lead roundhouse kick is a particularly effective quick kick because of your proximity to your opponent. This swift and powerful combative strike targets the opponent's vulnerable leg areas. The medium-height roundhouse kick targets the groin, midsection, ribs, and kidneys, whereas a high roundhouse kick targets the neck and head. From your left outlet stance, you will take a small 45-degree step with your right leg to begin to open up your hips for the kick. As you take the 45-degree step, raise your lead leg, rotating the knee, thigh, and shin parallel to the ground. Pivot on the ball of your base-leg foot so your body turns to the right, in the direction of your kneecap. (If your pivot is correct when you practice without a pad or bag, you will end up with your buttocks toward an imaginary opponent in front of you, having traced an imaginary arc with your foot.) Keep your eyes on your target. Continue to pivot and swing around toward your opponent as you straighten and strengthen your kicking leg to execute the kick. Notice from the photos that you are leaning back slightly.

As with your other combative strikes, your entire weight drives through the kick while your body torques through the target. When your body turns, keep your eyes on your target. As you kick, your hip must "roll over," or rotate parallel to the ground. Remember: as shown in the photos, you are leaning back somewhat, so your foot is parallel to the ground at the point of impact. You can increase the power and efficacy of this kick by shooting your same-side arm out at the opponent. This is not a strike so much as a directional and range finder that forces your body weight forward to further add to the kick's power. As you connect with your shin against the opponent, extend your toes, straighten your leg, and attack the Achilles, knee joint, thigh, or midsection. To avoid injury, do not strike with the top of your foot.

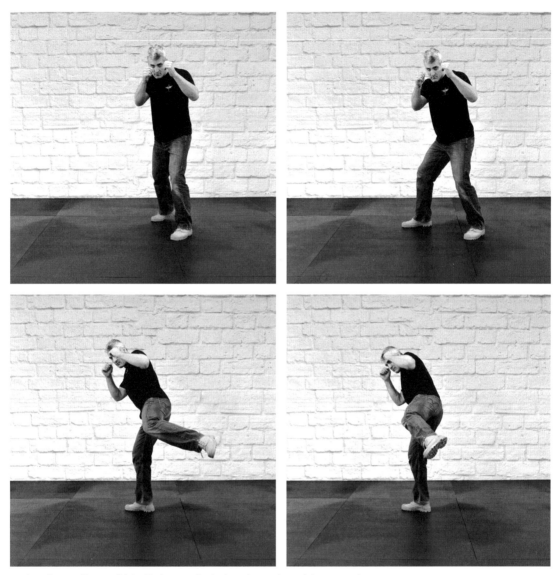

Lead roundhouse kick. Note rear foot stepping outward to generate power.

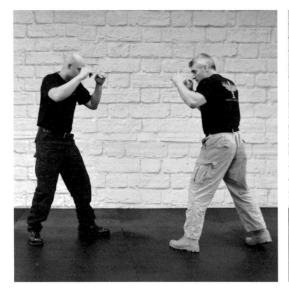
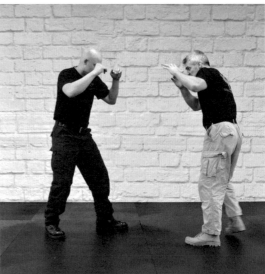

Lead roundhouse kick. Note rear foot stepping outward to generate power.

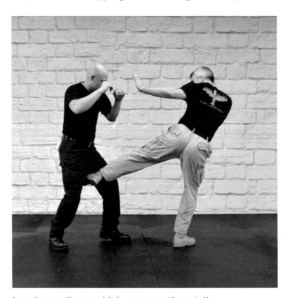

Lead roundhouse kick, preemptive strike.

Rear Roundhouse Kick

Similar to the lead roundhouse kick, the powerful rear roundhouse kick attacks the opponent's vulnerable leg areas. A medium-height roundhouse kick targets the groin, midsection, ribs, and kidneys, whereas a high roundhouse kick targets the neck and head. From your left outlet stance, raise your rear leg (similar to the beginning stage of a rear straight kick), and then rotate the knee, thigh, and shin parallel to the ground. Pivot on the ball of your base-leg foot so your body turns to the left, in the direction of your kneecap. (If your pivot is correct, when you practice without a pad or bag, you will end up with your buttocks toward an imaginary opponent in front of you, having traced an imaginary arc with your foot.) Keep your eyes on your target. Continue to pivot and swing around toward your opponent as you straighten and strengthen your kicking leg to execute the kick. As with your other combative strikes, your entire weight comes through the kick while your body torques through the target. When your body turns, keep your eyes on your target. As you kick, your hip must "roll over," or rotate parallel to the ground, so your foot is parallel to the ground. Again, you are leaning back slightly. You can increase the power and efficacy of this kick by shooting your same-side arm out at the opponent. This is not a strike so much as a direction and range finder that forces your body weight forward to further add to the kick's power. Notice in the photos the significant turn of the base leg—as much as 90 degrees or more.

You can connect with either your shin or with the ball of your foot. To avoid injury, do not strike with the top of your foot. If you use your shin, extend your toes, straighten your leg, and attack the Achilles, knee joint, thigh, or midsection. If you choose to connect with the ball of your foot, pull the toes back and keep your foot parallel to the ground. This second option provides a more precise striking surface, ideal for striking the groin. To facilitate the kick and accelerate the pivot, you can also take a step out with the base leg to set up the roundhouse kick rather than spinning on the ball of your foot. This shortcut is particularly useful for low, powerful sweeps against an attacker's Achilles. Note: You can easily convert a roundhouse shin kick into a sweep by lowering your center of gravity to target the opponent's Achilles tendon just above the ankle.

What to Do If Your Opponent Catches Your Leg

If you have thrown a lead or rear roundhouse kick and your opponent catches your leg, immediately close the distance to your opponent by bending the knee of your caught leg. Counterattack as soon as possible with eye gouges, strikes, or execute a jumping clinch by grabbing the opponent's head to position your body to defend a takedown.

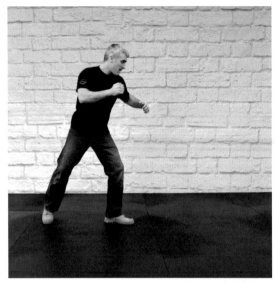 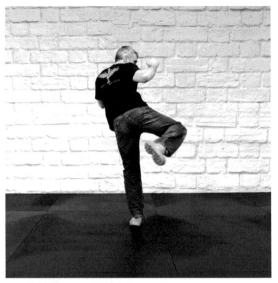

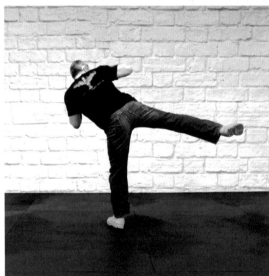

Rear roundhouse kick. Note full pivot on the ball of the foot, base leg.

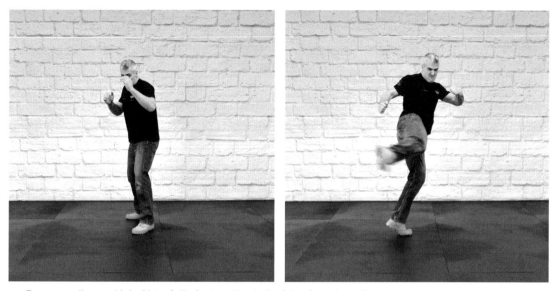

Rear roundhouse kick. Note full pivot on the ball of the foot, base leg.

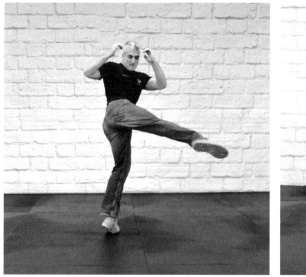

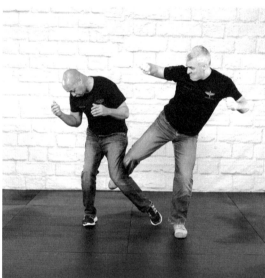

Rear roundhouse kick targeting the thigh or knee.

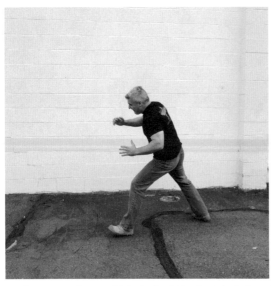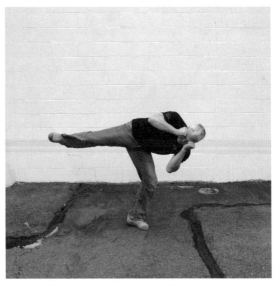

Rear roundhouse kick, ball-of-the-foot variation. Note base-leg pivot combined with body defense. This kick can be used to deliver a groin strike to someone who is in a bladed stance.

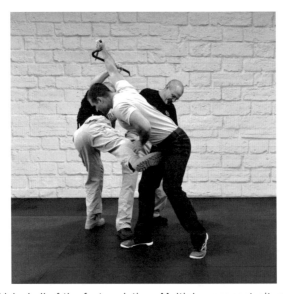

Rear roundhouse kick, ball-of-the-foot variation. Multiple-opponent situation. Note base-leg pivot combined with body defense.

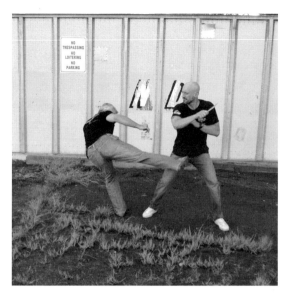

Rear roundhouse kick, ball-of-the-foot variation in defending an edged-weapon backslash. Note base-leg pivot combined with body defense.

Low Roundhouse Kick Sweep

The low roundhouse kick sweep buckles or "sweeps" an opponent's leg or legs out. The main target is usually the Achilles tendon; however, the knees are also vulnerable to this type of combative. To deliver the low roundhouse kick sweep from your left outlet stance, raise your rear leg and then rotate the knee, thigh, and shin parallel to the ground. Pivot on the ball of your base-leg foot while bending the knee slightly, so your body turns to the left in the direction of your kneecap. When you bend the knee, your leg will necessarily extend out farther to facilitate sweeping your opponent. Keep your eyes on your target. Continue to pivot and swing around toward your opponent as you straighten and strengthen your kicking leg to kick through him. As with your other combative strikes, your entire weight comes through the kick while your body torques through the target like a hatchet chopping down a tree. As your body turns, keep your eyes on your target. When you kick sweep, your hip must rotate parallel, forcing you to lean back slightly. Lower your center of gravity to target the opponent's Achilles tendon just above the ankle.

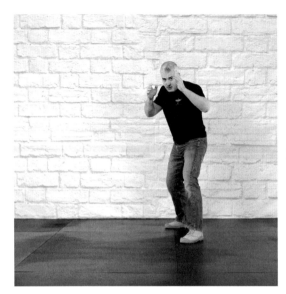
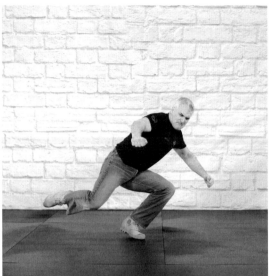
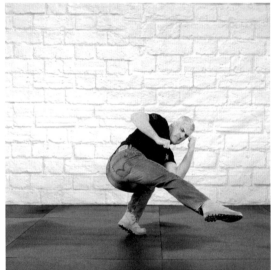

Low roundhouse kick sweep. Note the base-leg pivot.

Roundhouse Kick from the Ground

A roundhouse kick can also be effectively delivered should you find yourself on the ground, facing a standing opponent. To deliver the kick you must rise off the ground, either by using two hands to lift your torso, or, alternatively, using a forearm to lift your body. As you lift yourself from the ground, your base leg must pivot—as with all kicks— to allow your hips to fully engage throughout the kick and place your body weight behind it. It is also possible with upper-body strength and athletic prowess to raise your entire body off the ground and swivel your entire torso into the opponent. Contact is made with your shin against the opponent's knee or thigh.

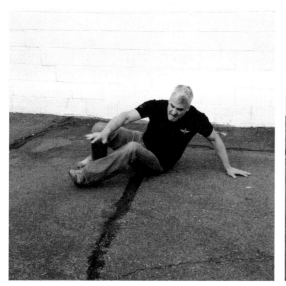
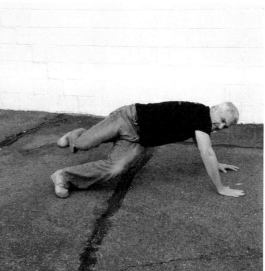

Roundhouse kick from the ground. Note body raise for maximum reach and power.

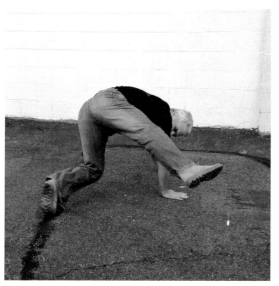
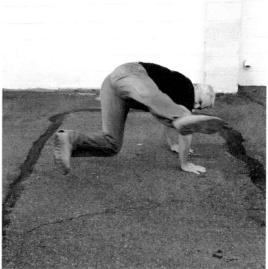

Roundhouse kick from the ground, two variations. First photo: pivot foot on ground. Second photo: only hands on ground, no pivot foot. Note body raise for maximum reach and power.

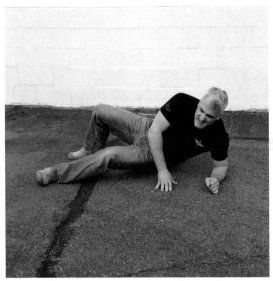
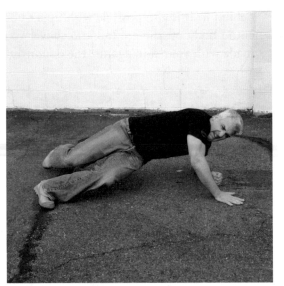
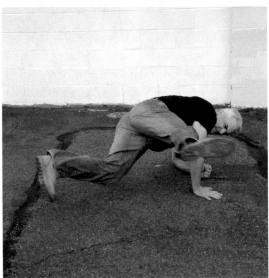

Roundhouse kick from the ground, forearm-pivot variation. Note body raise for maximum reach and power.

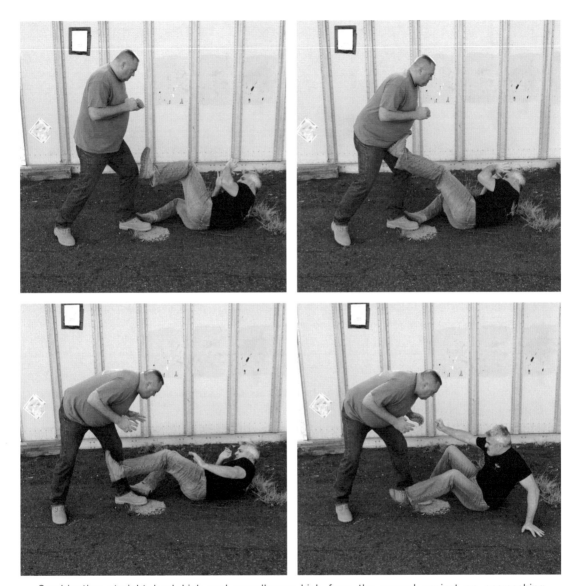

Combination straight heel kick and roundhouse kick from the ground against an encroaching opponent.

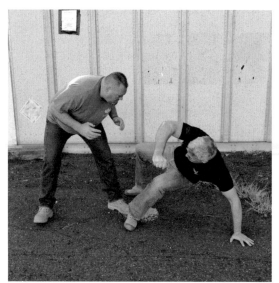 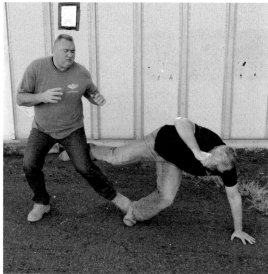

Combination straight heel kick and roundhouse kick from the ground against an encroaching opponent. Note body raise for maximum reach and power.

Rear Roundhouse Knee

Similar to a roundhouse kick, this best targets the kidneys and ribs. Use the same technique and movement for the lead and rear roundhouse knees as you do for the lead and rear roundhouse kicks, except do not extend your leg. Instead, you will connect with your kneecap rather than your foot. Always keep your hands up as you move. Notice in the photos the significant turn of the base leg. In the depicted punch defense, the defender recognizes an attempted sucker punch and instinctively uses a 360 outside defense (deflection) combined with a roundhouse-knee counterattack to the attacker's kidneys.

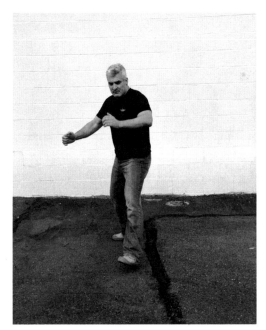 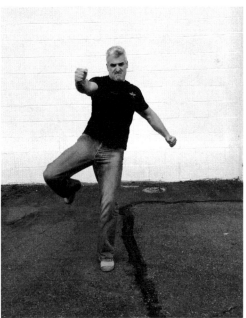

Rear roundhouse knee.

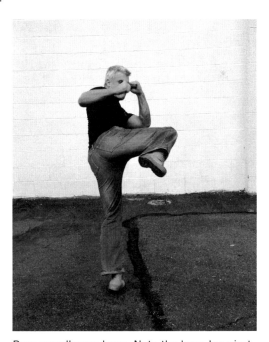

Rear roundhouse knee. Note the base-leg pivot.

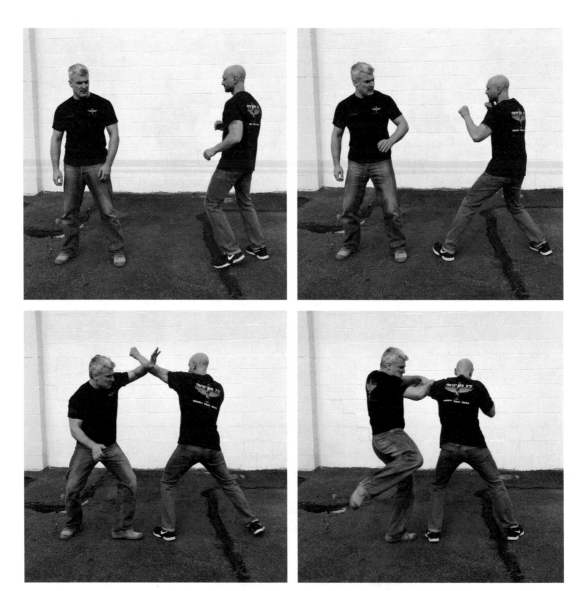

A 360 outside deflection combined with a rear roundhouse knee in defending a sucker punch. Note the base-leg pivot.

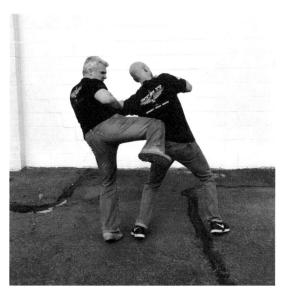

A 360 outside deflection combined with a rear roundhouse knee in defending a sucker punch.

Rear Half-Roundhouse Knee

The rear half-roundhouse knee utilizes both the shinbone and the patella to make contact with the opponent's thigh. As with all kicks and knee strikes, your base leg pivots to allow your hips full follow-through for maximum power.

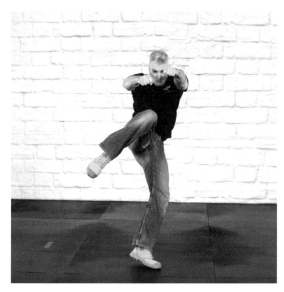

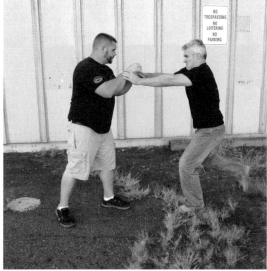

Rear half-roundhouse knee with arm-trap option.

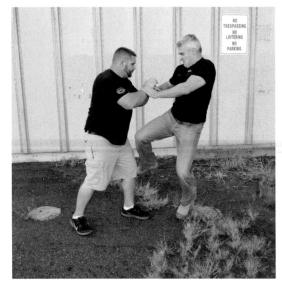 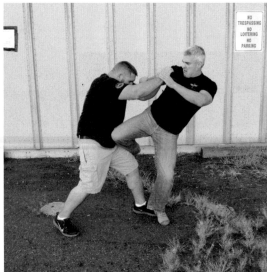

Rear half-roundhouse knee with arm-trap option. Note the base-leg pivot.

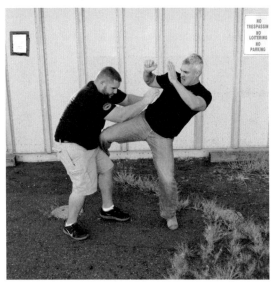 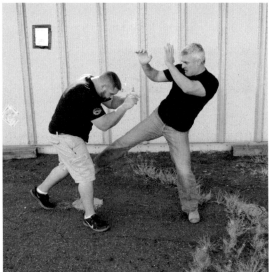

Roundhouse knee with arm-trap option.

CHAPTER 5

Combatives Combinations and Retzev

Kick Combinations

Combination kicks allow a defender to use the lower body's powerful muscles and reach to debilitate an attacker. Targets usually include the knee, thigh, and groin. Of course, targets higher on the body are also available, including the stomach, solar plexus, chin, and face. The following four kick combinations are highly effective:

1. Lead straight kick into rear straight kick (using opposite legs)
2. Rear straight kick into rear straight kick (using opposite legs by having the rear kick land forward and making the former lead leg the rear leg)
3. Lead straight kick into rear roundhouse kick (using opposite legs)
4. Lead roundhouse kick into rear roundhouse kick (using opposite legs)

Note: As an opening salvo, we prefer to use a lead roundhouse kick rather than a rear roundhouse kick. A rear roundhouse kick momentarily exposes the groin to counterattack by virtue of the kicking motion and the longer time a rear kick takes to reach the target.

Kick and Knee Combinations

Kicks may also be combined with knee strikes, if one's first kick does not drive the opponent back. The following five kick and knee combinations are highly effective:

1. Straight-kick combination into same-leg straight knee strike
2. Lead straight kick into rear straight knee (using opposite legs)
3. Rear straight kick into rear straight knee (using opposite legs by having the rear kick landing forward, thus switching lead legs)

4. Rear straight knee into rear straight knee (using opposite legs by having the rear knee landing forward, thus switching lead legs)

5. Lead roundhouse kick into rear straight kick (using opposite legs)

Straight Kick and Straight Knee Combinations

Straight Kick into Same-Leg Straight Knee Strike

This combination delivers a long-range straight kick to an opponent's groin or midsection, thereby buckling or bending him forward. As you have reduced the opponent's level down, you can target the head with a knee strike, using the same leg as you delivered in the longer-range straight kick. As your straight kick touches down, use a shuffle step with your rear leg to replace your lead leg, enabling you to strike the opponent in the head with your knee.

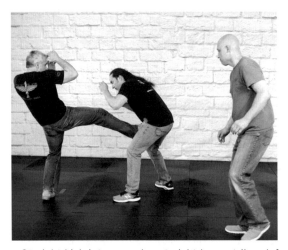 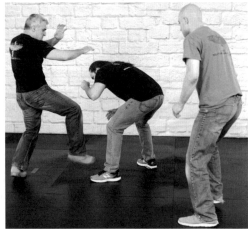

Straight kick into same-leg straight knee strike, defending against multiple opponents.

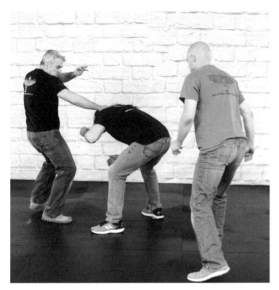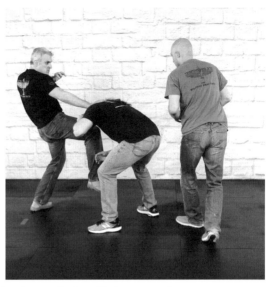

Straight kick into same-leg straight knee strike, defending against multiple opponents.

Rear Straight Knee Rechambering

Rechambering a rear straight knee—bringing the knee strike into its original position—delivers a strong, debilitating combative combination. Be sure to pivot on the base leg for maximum reach and power for each successive knee strike. After each knee strike, draw your knee back to the rear in its original position. This rear position cocks your hip and knee to deliver a powerful strike. Be sure to drive *through* the target with your patella, not upward. Note: An upward knee to the face is devastating but follows a different trajectory, as incorporated into the different defenses found in the vertical elbow drop strike #5 photo series.

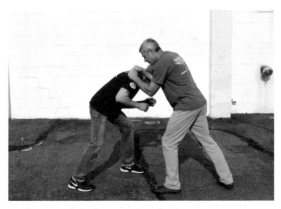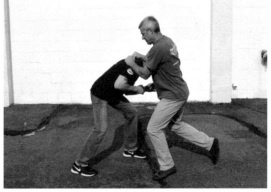

Rear straight knee rechambering

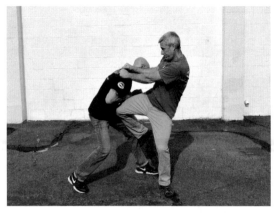 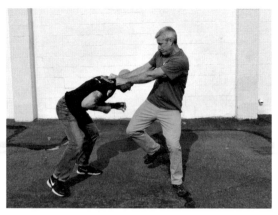

Rear straight knee rechambering. Note the base-leg pivot.

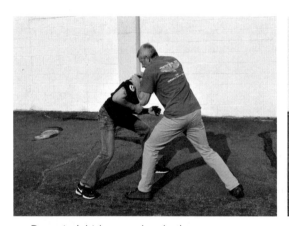 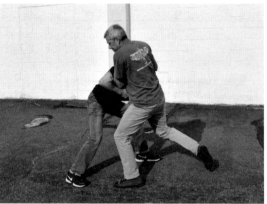

Rear straight knee rechambering.

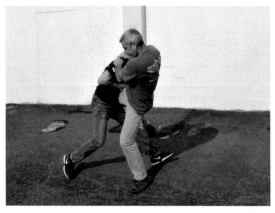

Rear straight knee rechambering. Note the base-leg pivot.

Compound Kick Combinations

Compound kicks using the same kicking leg epitomize economy of motion by harnessing the momentum from one kick and using it instantaneously to launch another kick. Compound kicks require both balance and strength. The key is to avoid touching your kicking leg to the ground. Of course, while you can set the kicking leg down, this interrupts the economy of motion because you then need to rechamber to deliver the kick. This touchdown of your kicking leg, while it too can be effective, may upset the timing of a subsequent kick, as the opponent's vulnerable targeted anatomy may no longer be available.

Straight Kick into Side Kick

A straight kick may be followed immediately by using the same kicking leg to deliver a devastating side kick to an attacker's knee. This combination same-leg kick harnesses the straight kick's power and natural "bounceback" from the strong contact it makes with an attacker's groin or torso. As soon as the kick makes contact, the kravist continues to move his base foot. This facilitates a further pivot to allow an optimum side kick. Note: The straight kick into this combination kick is best delivered from the rear leg.

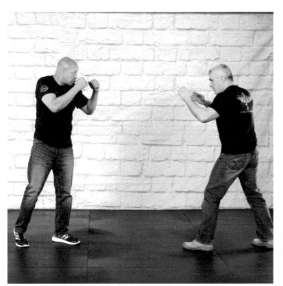 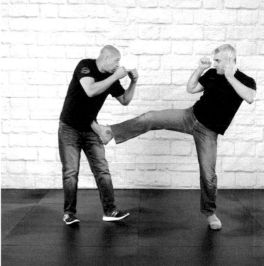

Straight kick into side kick. Note the base-leg pivot.

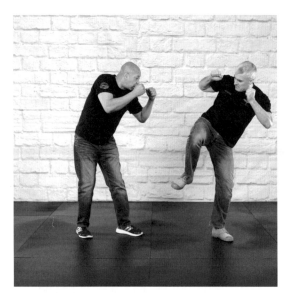 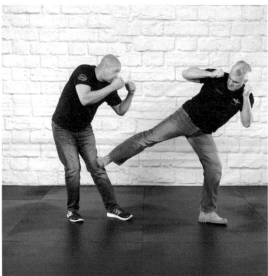

Straight kick into side kick. Note the base-leg pivot.

Lead Roundhouse Kick into Side Kick

A lead roundhouse kick against an opponent's lead leg may be followed immediately using the same kicking leg to deliver a devastating side kick to the opponent's rear knee. This combination same-leg kick harnesses the lead roundhouse kick's power and natural "bounce-back" from the strong contact it makes with an attacker's targeted leg. As soon as the lead roundhouse kick makes contact with the opponent's lead leg, continue to move your base foot, further pivoting to allow an optimum side kick to his opposite knee. Note: The lead roundhouse kick may target the opponent's inner thigh or his lead knee. If you buckle the opponent's lead knee with an initial lead roundhouse kick, there may not be an opportunity to deliver the follow-up side kick; however, the opponent is likely to go down, thereby presenting other combative opportunities. For example, you may immediately follow this lead roundhouse with an additional kick, using the same kicking leg. You could use the ball or the top of your foot or, alternatively, the shin, to deliver a straight kick (not depicted) to the opponent's groin.

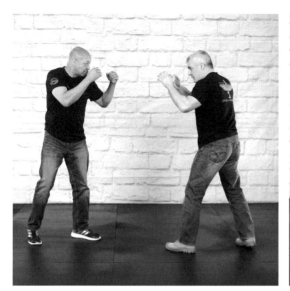
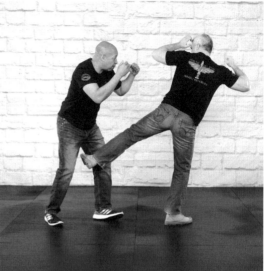
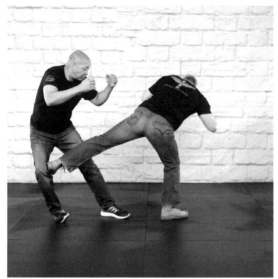

Lead roundhouse kick into side kick. Note rear foot outside step for reach and power.

Lead Roundhouse Kick into Ankle Stomp

A lead roundhouse kick may buckle an opponent's lead leg, sending him to the ground. If the kick is powerful enough, it may drop the opponent immediately, allowing for a devastating follow-up stomp to the opponent's exposed Achilles tendon or ankle.

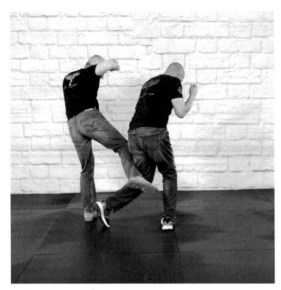
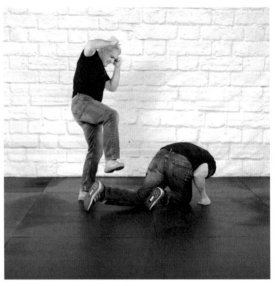

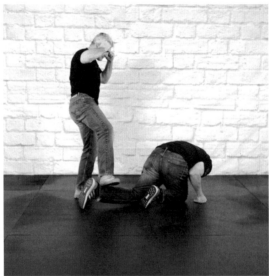

Lead roundhouse kick into ankle stomp.

Knee and Elbow Combinations

Knee and elbow combinations unleash some of your most powerful combatives when in close quarters. While they are short-range combatives, each strike requires long movement, or maximum reach, combined with full hip extensions and correct pivoting on the balls of your feet. A straight knee strike naturally leads to an elbow-strike option (including elbows #1, #4, and #8) as the body weight shifts forward onto the front pivot leg, allowing the opposite leg to immediately deliver a straight knee strike. Conversely, an elbow-strike option (including elbows #1, #4, and #8) naturally leads to a straight knee strike. The body weight shifts forward, delivering the elbow strike as the leg that delivered the straight knee strike touches down to the ground.

Lead Horizontal and Rear Horizontal Elbow Combination

This lead horizontal and rear horizontal elbow one-two combination takes advantage of the momentum of your body movement. This combination is a great tactic to launch into retzev. Begin in your left outlet stance with your hands protecting your face. Deliver a lead horizontal elbow strike. As soon as you reach your maximum left pivot, immediately follow up with a rear horizontal strike. You can also deliver the horizontal elbow strike from a crouch.

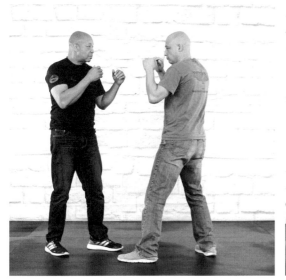 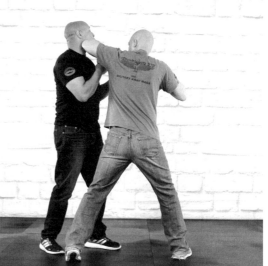

Lead and rear horizontal elbow combination. Note full pivot to the right.

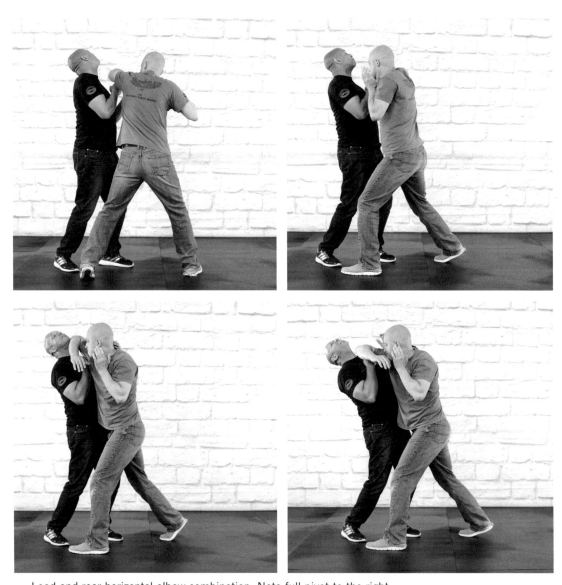

Lead and rear horizontal elbow combination. Note full pivot to the right.

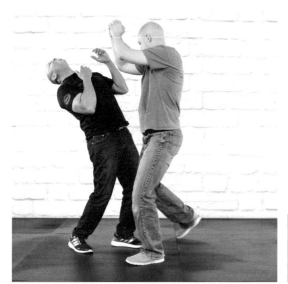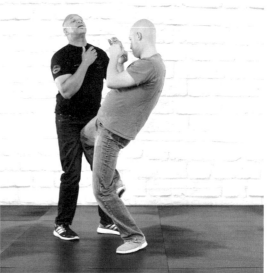

Lead and rear horizontal elbow combination. Note full pivot to the right.

Rear Knee Followed by Horizontal Elbow and Uppercut Elbow Combination

This combination takes advantage of the momentum of your body movement. It is a great tactic to launch into close-quarters retzev. Begin in your left outlet stance with your hands protecting your face. Deliver a rear straight knee strike. As you begin to touch down with your right foot—you are now in a right outlet stance—launch a lead horizontal elbow strike #1 (with your right elbow), making sure to use maximum reach. Follow through completely and then execute a rear uppercut elbow strike #4 with your left arm. This is followed by a rear straight knee. Note how on your rear uppercut #4 elbow strike, your weight shifted to your lead leg as you pivoted. This weight shift facilitates the movement of your rear left leg into a straight knee strike.

Note that you can also omit the knee strike for a variation of this technique. To do so, begin in your left outlet stance. You will deliver a lead horizontal elbow and a rear uppercut elbow—a "one-two" combination that takes advantage of the momentum of your body movement. This combination is a great tactic to launch into retzev. Begin in your left outlet stance with your hands protecting your face. Deliver a lead horizontal elbow strike. As soon as you reach your maximum left pivot, immediately follow up with a rear uppercut elbow strike. Again, you can also deliver the horizontal and uppercut elbow strikes from a crouch.

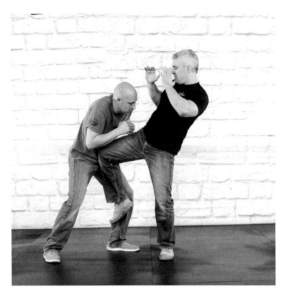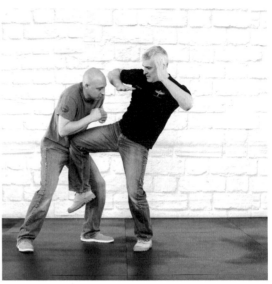

Rear knee and horizontal uppercut elbow combination. Note the base-leg pivot.

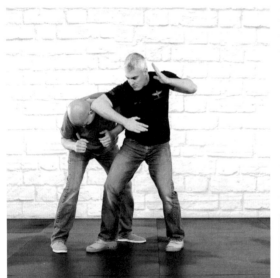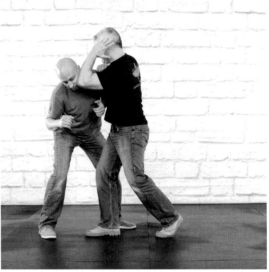

Rear knee and horizontal uppercut elbow combination. Note full left pivot and uppercut pivot.

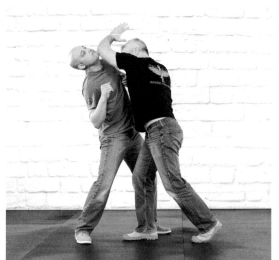 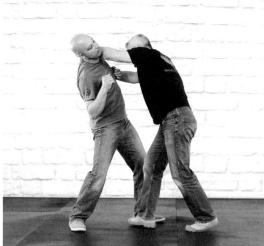

Rear knee and horizontal uppercut elbow combination.

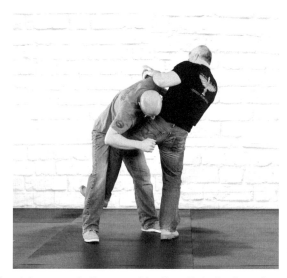

Rear knee and horizontal uppercut elbow combination. Note the base-leg pivot.

Hand Groin Smash and Uppercut Elbow Strike #7 Combination

A hand groin smash can be combined with an uppercut elbow strike #7 to debilitate an opponent. The hand groin smash will likely double over the opponent, allowing you to use an immediate uppercut #7 elbow strike to the opponent's chin. Be sure to cock your hips and shoot upward by straightening your legs, exploding into the opponent's jaw with the elbow strike.

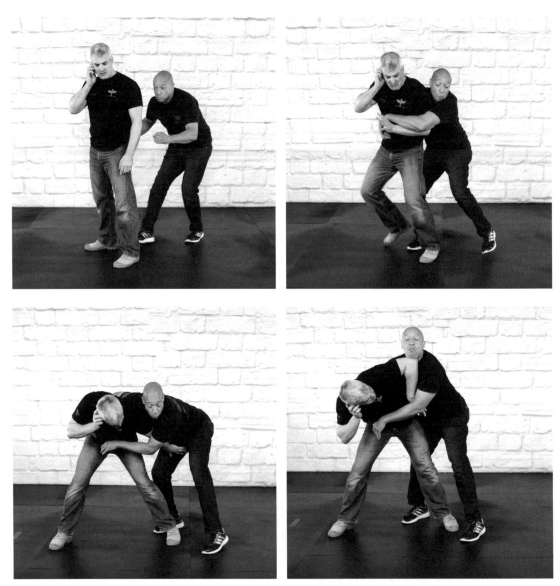

Hand groin smash and uppercut elbow strike #7 combination used in defending a rear bear-hug attempt.

Chop Combinations

A double chop combination using an outside chop followed by an inside chop is a highly effective method of rendering an opponent unconscious. Even if the opponent is not rendered unconscious, the strike can inflict momentary, debilitating pain. A correctly placed chop to the carotid sinus interrupts the blood flow to the brain, thereby tampering with an opponent's blood pressure and vascular tone. If you deliver a double chop to the carotid, it haywires the opponent's brain even more, temporarily shutting down his system and causing unconsciousness. The vagus nerve, which plays a central role in the body's involuntary nervous system, may also be struck, resulting in disorientation, temporary blindness, dizziness, or a brief loss of consciousness.

Lead and Rear Chop Combination

A highly effective combination involves an outside chop followed by an immediate inside chop targeting the same anatomy point.

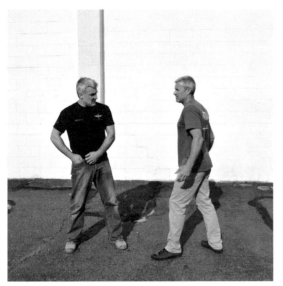 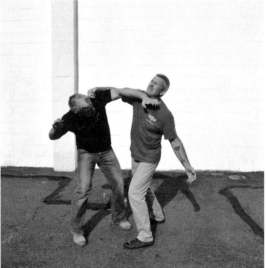

Lead and rear chop combination preemption defending a hook punch.

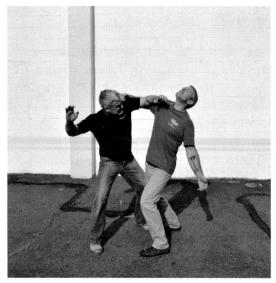 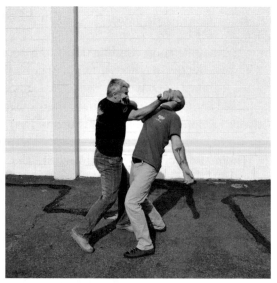

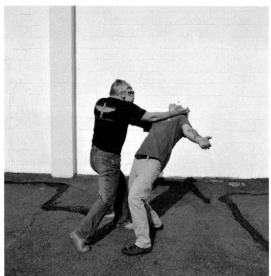

Lead and rear chop combination preemption defending a hook punch.

Kick-and-Punch Combinations

Kick-and-punch combinations are the backbone of retzev when combined with other strikes. The key is to deliver the punch just as the kicking foot is landing, to harness the body's power through the punch without having to take an additional step—a good example of krav maga's emphasis on economy of motion.

Straight Lead Shuffle Kick into Two Straight Punches Followed by Rear Roundhouse Kick

The straight lead shuffle kick into two straight punches followed by a roundhouse kick is a powerful linear combination of straight kicks and punches. The key is delivering a mechanically sound straight lead shuffle kick by moving your rear foot forward to replace where your front foot was. This shuffle moves your entire body weight through the kick. As you touch down with the kicking foot, deliver the lead straight punch, transferring your weight onto your lead leg as you connect with the straight punch. This lead straight punch sets up a rear straight punch, as your weight can easily transfer from your rear leg to pivot through the straight punch. As you pivot through your straight punch, your weight remains on your lead leg and the ball of the foot of your rear leg. Pivoting on the ball of the foot facilitates a strong rear roundhouse kick.

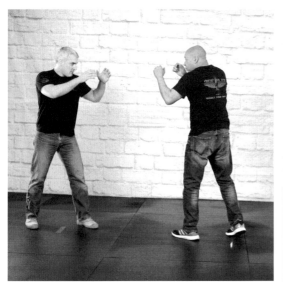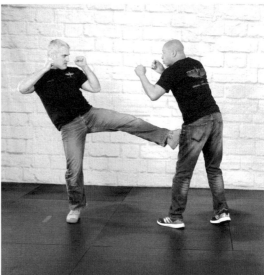

Straight lead kick → two straight punches → rear roundhouse kick → heel stomp.

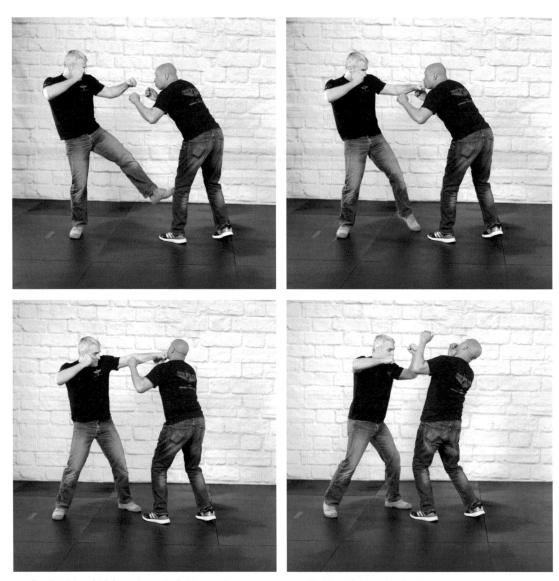

Straight lead kick → two straight punches → rear roundhouse kick → heel stomp.

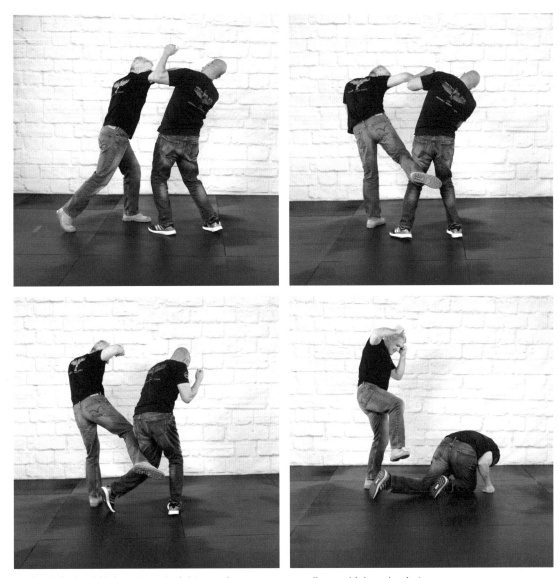

Straight lead kick → two straight punches → rear roundhouse kick → heel stomp.

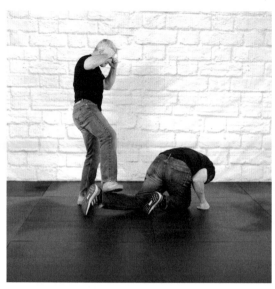

Straight lead kick → two straight punches → rear roundhouse kick → heel stomp.

Lead Roundhouse Kick into Two Straight Punches Followed by Roundhouse Kick

This is another powerful kick-and-punch combination. A roundhouse kick delivered with the shin places you in precise punching range. Once again, the key is delivering a technically sound lead roundhouse kick. As you touch down with the kicking foot to deliver the lead straight punch, transfer your weight onto your lead leg as you connect with the lead straight punch. This lead straight punch sets up a strong subsequent rear straight punch, as your weight can easily transfer from your rear leg to pivot through the straight punch. As you pivot through your straight punch, your weight remains on your lead leg and ball of the foot of your rear leg. The ball-of-the-foot pivot on the rear leg facilitates a strong rear roundhouse kick.

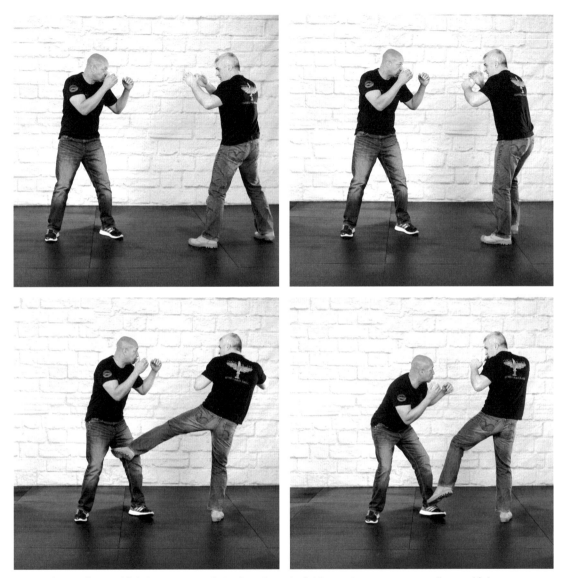

Lead roundhouse kick (note outward step) → two straight punches → rear roundhouse kick.

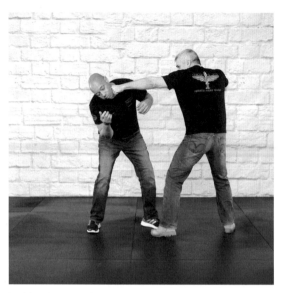

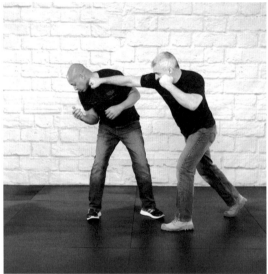
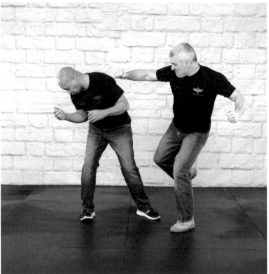

Lead roundhouse kick (note outward step) → two straight punches → rear roundhouse kick.

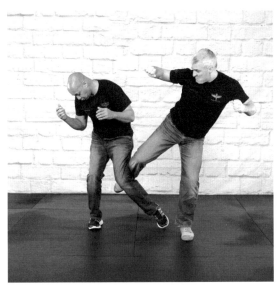

Lead roundhouse kick (note outward step) → two straight punches → rear roundhouse kick (note base-leg pivot).

Hammer Fist, Knee, and Elbow Combinations

The following examples show a combination of upper-body and lower-body short-range strikes similar in concept to the previous long- and medium-range kick-and-punch combinations. One strike leads into another practical, opportune strike, harnessing the striker's momentum that undergirds economy of motion.

Straight Knee Strike into Vertical Elbow Drop Strike #5

A knee strike to the stomach, groin, or thigh that doubles an opponent over sets up a vertical elbow drop #5 (or hammer-fist strike, as the next example provides) to the back of the opponent's neck, his kidneys, or other vulnerable anatomy. The key is dropping the vertical elbow strike #5 as the kneeing leg touches down. This timing and coordination optimizes the strike by delivering all of the defender's body weight down through the strike. This epitomizes krav maga's economy of motion concept. Note: You will see this combination again in the first retzev example below.

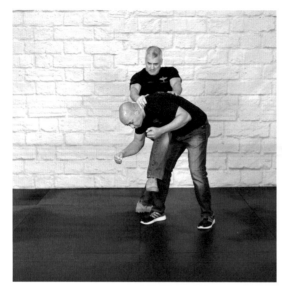 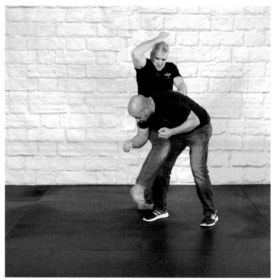

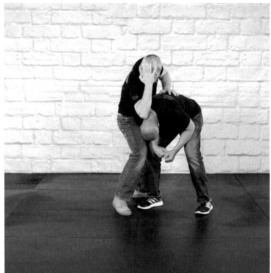

Straight knee strike into vertical elbow strike #5.

Retzev—The Force Multiplier: Untamed, Targeted, Continuous Counterviolence

Forming the backbone of the Israeli fighting system, retzev is a seamless, decisive, and overwhelming counterattack. In short, you will launch an untamed response, using optimized strikes, takedowns, throws, joint locks, chokes, or other offensive actions, combined with evasive action. Israeli krav maga taught by Grandmaster Haim Gidon uses retzev ("continuous combat motion") to overpower an assailant and complete the defense. In his last years, Imi spoke of the retzev concept. Haim understood and implemented it. The top Gidon krav maga students are known for their ability to execute retzev.

An analogy for retzev might be a well-placed bullet from a semiautomatic weapon followed by that weapon's then going fully automatic to finish the threat. Key retzev principles are as follows:

- There are no preconceived routines or sets of combatives; however, there are logical combinations of combatives built into your personal retzev to take advantage of anatomical targets of opportunity.

- Retzev teaches the defender to move instinctively in combat motion *without thinking* about the next logical move.

- Retzev, armed or unarmed, is quick and decisive movement merging all aspects of one's krav maga training.

- Defensive movements transition automatically and seamlessly into offensive movements to neutralize the attack, leaving an adversary little or no time to react.

- If attacked, the kravist must—within the boundaries of the law—become the most viscerally violent person present, capable of defeating any threat.

Retzev may be compared to a professional law enforcement or military assault. Professional military and law enforcement personnel use overwhelming violence of action and a preponderance of firepower; criminals try to do the same.

In the following examples of partial retzev, you will see simulations of this *untamed, targeted, continuous counterviolence*. Note that the defender preempts the opponent's aggressive movement or immediately takes the fight to him when the opponent displays a fighting stance.

Retzev Example #1

This first retzev example shows a continuous flow of combatives that is initiated with a lead side kick followed immediately by a lead hammer-fist strike. The defender preempts the opponent's attack by delivering a right side kick to the opponent's knee followed by a right hammer-fist strike. You will note that the right hammer-fist punch is delivered as the kicking leg touches down, thereby transferring one's body weight forward to harness momentum and drive one's body mass through the target. This is one of retzev's essential tenets, along with logical, instinctive movements. The right hammer-fist strike transfers one's weight to the lead leg, thus allowing a left rear straight punch. The left rear straight punch, in turn, transfers weight onto the lead leg, facilitating a left half-roundhouse knee to the opponent's nearside thigh. As the left half-roundhouse knee makes impact, body weight is again transferred forward, allowing for a right inside chop to the opponent's kidneys. The inside chop is delivered as the lead leg touches down once again, harnessing weight transfer to the lead leg. This in turn facilitates a right rear straight knee strike to the opponent's head. Because the weight is loaded on the rear leg, the lead leg may readily deliver the final side kick to the opponent's knee to put him on the ground. Importantly, while this example shows retzev's continuous flow of combatives, if any one of the combatives is decisive in felling the opponent, thereby stopping the threat, the defender must cease his counteroffensive actions or he risks using excessive force. In other words, a self-defense claim will no longer be valid if you continue to gratuitously beat and injure an erstwhile attacker.

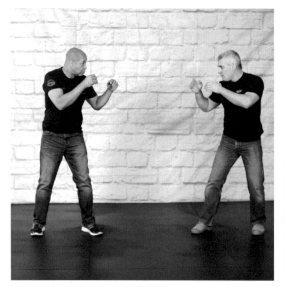 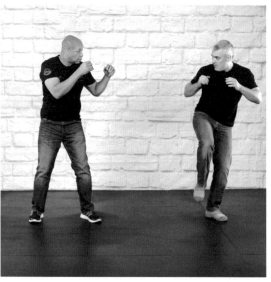

Retzev: right side kick → right backfist → left straight punch → left half-roundhouse knee → right chop → right straight knee → right side kick.

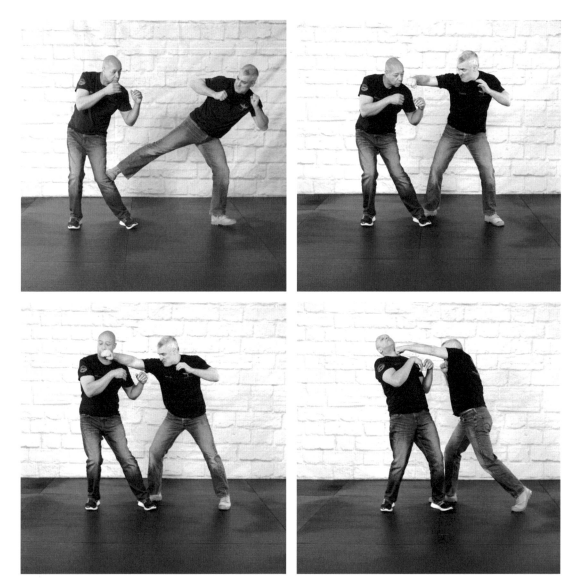

Retzev: right side kick → right backfist → left straight punch → left half-roundhouse knee → right chop → right straight knee → right side kick.

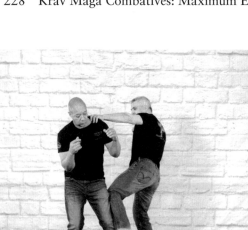
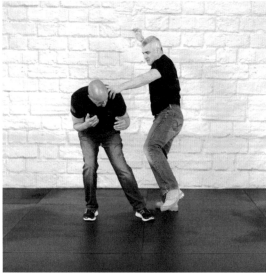
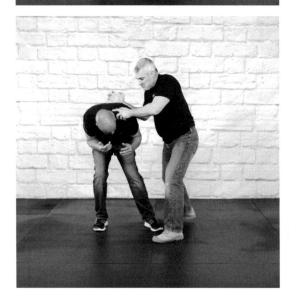
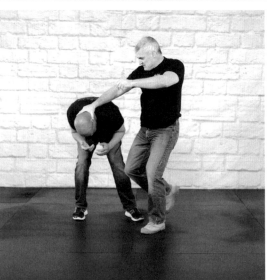

Retzev: right side kick → right backfist → left straight punch → left half-roundhouse knee → right chop → right straight knee → right side kick.

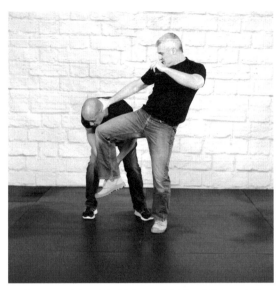 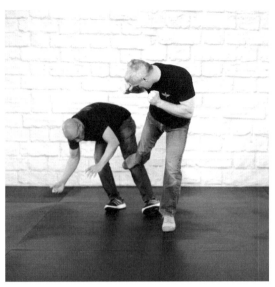

Retzev: right side kick → right backfist → left straight punch → left half-roundhouse knee → right chop → right straight knee → right side kick.

Retzev Example #2 against Concerted Resistance

Similar to retzev example #1, this second retzev example shows a preemptive lead straight kick to the opponent's groin, followed by a straight-punch left-right combination and a half-roundhouse knee strike. Notwithstanding the defender's strong combatives, the adversary continues his attack. Importantly, this example demonstrates an opponent sustaining damage but still continuing to attack you. As noted previously, understanding that an opponent will continue to attack you is a hallmark of any good self-defense training. *The opponent is not going to cooperate with your counterattack.* Accordingly, the defender is executing his counterattack while simultaneously defending against the opponent's attempt to keep fighting. Therefore, retzev must always be adjusted on the fly and instinctively to orchestrate a continuous-motion counterattack while maintaining the ability to defend. Obviously, the time-honored adage that the best defense is a good offense is evident.

In continuing the counterattack, following the half-hook punch, the defender uses a modified lead half-roundhouse knee strike against the opponent's midsection. Despite absorbing a lead half-roundhouse knee to the midsection, the opponent continues to fight back by attempting a hook punch. The defender reacts instinctively with a double forearm block against the opponent's right hook punch, followed immediately by a right outside chop to the opponent's right carotid artery. After temporarily stunning the opponent, the defender seizes the opportunity to deliver a nearside right straight knee to the opponent's head followed by a police control hold #6 (also known as *kimura*) to finally control the opponent and summon the police.

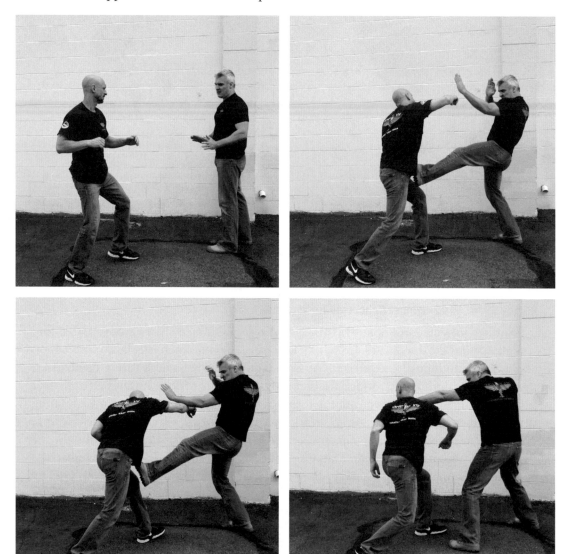

Retzev: straight left groin kick → straight left punch → right half-roundhouse punch → left half-roundhouse knee strike → right outside chop → nearside right straight knee → kimura hold (police control #6).

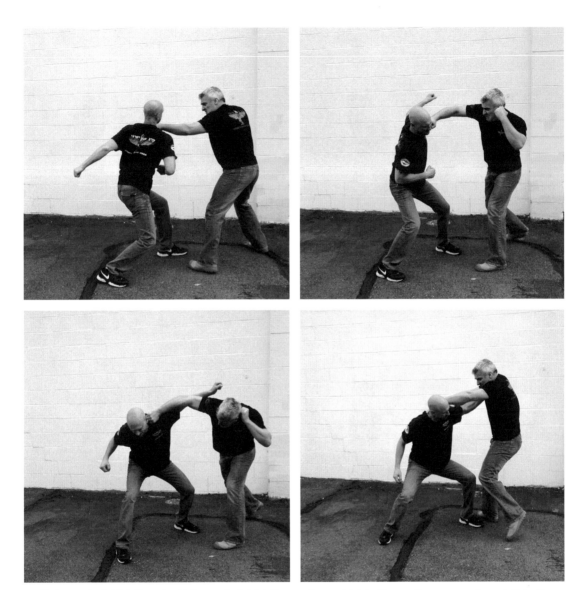

Retzev: straight left groin kick → straight left punch → right half-roundhouse punch → left half-roundhouse knee strike → right outside chop → nearside right straight knee → kimura hold (police control #6).

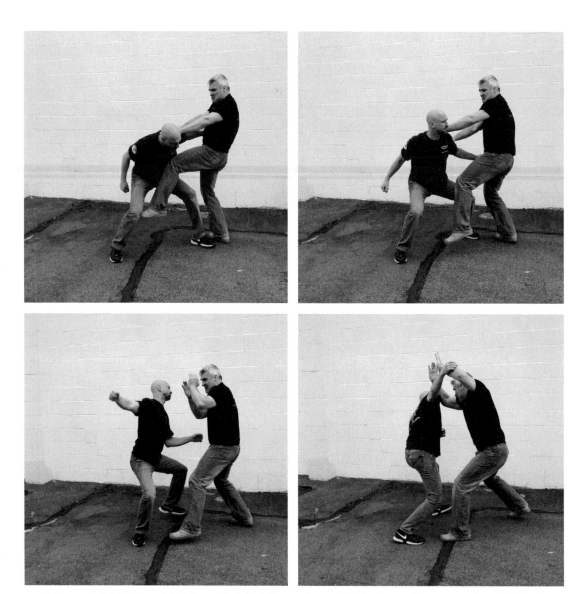

Retzev: straight left groin kick → straight left punch → right half-roundhouse punch → left half-roundhouse knee strike → right outside chop → nearside right straight knee → kimura hold (police control #6).

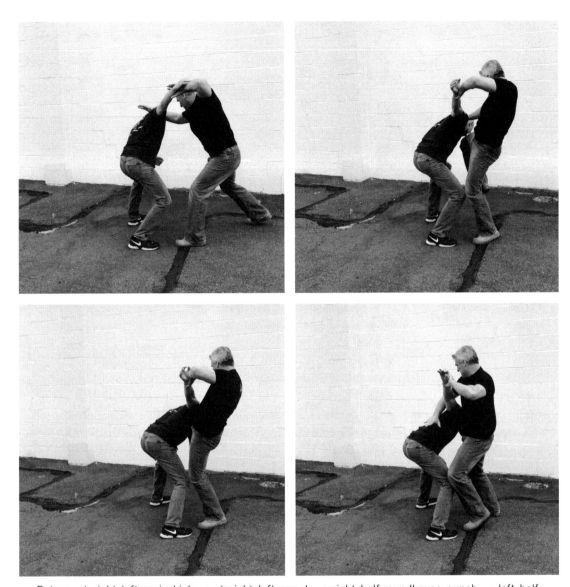

Retzev: straight left groin kick → straight left punch → right half-roundhouse punch → left half-roundhouse knee strike → right outside chop → nearside right straight knee → kimura hold (police control #6).

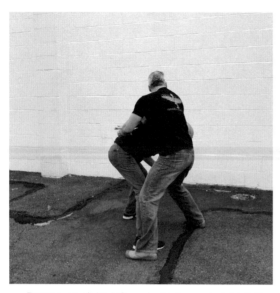 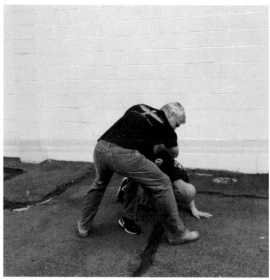

Retzev: straight left groin kick → straight left punch → right half-roundhouse punch → left half-roundhouse knee strike → right outside chop → nearside right straight knee → kimura hold (police control #6). Then summon the police.

As noted, the reader may wonder how an opponent could withstand such a counter-attack using strong, targeted combatives. There are individuals who can withstand enormous thresholds of physical punishment and keep on fighting. This is especially true if the opponent is under the influence of pain-numbing or adrenalizing narcotics.

CHAPTER 6
Takedowns and Throws

Combatives Family #11: Takedowns and Throws

The Israeli krav maga curriculum incorporates several core takedowns and throws. Founder Imi Lichtenfeld was awarded a black belt in judo through Moshe Feldenkrais, who trained in Japan directly under the legendary Kano Jigoro. For the green-belt level (third belt level in the official krav maga curriculum), Imi incorporated several of judo's most accessible and effective takedowns and throws. In choosing these takedowns and throws, Imi married the techniques with many of the core defenses against upper-body attacks. Imi recognized that by letting gravity take its course, coupled with momentum generated by the throw or takedown, slamming someone into the ground would help take the fight out of him—or, at the least, momentarily diminish his offensive capabilities.

Krav maga teaches simple and effective takedowns that usually flow naturally from other techniques to put an opponent on the ground. Think of these techniques as extensions of a previously completed combative technique, such as a gouge to the eyes to disorient an opponent while you perform an outside reverse sweep (osoto gari), as described below. Although more advanced hip throws and other takedowns are an integral part of advanced krav maga training, they are beyond the scope of this core krav maga combatives book.

Selecting a throw is generally determined by body positioning and the dynamics of the entry to the throw. The goal with throws and takedowns, as with all krav maga thinking, is to accomplish the greatest effect with the least effort.

Your aim in any type of takedown or throw is to ruin the opponent's balance while hastening his impact with the ground. In other words, undercut your adversary's balance by collapsing his structure. Tactically, this could include crippling one of his knees, sweeping his feet from under him, or picking him up and dropping him pointedly on a specific part of his anatomy. In short, krav maga takedowns and throws principally distill into two methods: (1) removing the opponent's base balance (his legs) or (2) forcing his center of gravity, which is just below the navel for most people, beyond a stable base (two balanced legs).

This type of combative that forces the opponent to drop unassisted or pounds him into the ground is designed to inflict serious damage such as a neck injury or spinal injury; skull fracture; broken wrist, elbow, or coccyx; damaged shoulder; or concussion. So, obviously, use this type of combative only when necessary. (Keep in mind, it is highly foreseeable that, if you trip or throw someone to the ground, a jury will conclude that you intended to seriously injure him.) Obviously, in a life-and-death violent encounter, you may wish to make the throw as damaging as possible. With a throw or takedown, physics dictates that you can heighten an impact's velocity by approximately 50 percent by undercutting both the opponent's legs from the ground as opposed to just one leg. While you can also maximize impact by adding your body weight to fall on top of the opponent, krav maga emphasizes remaining standing and mobile whenever possible.

For hip throws, your primary maneuverability and power come from your legs. As you enter the throw, the goal is to displace the adversary's base with your own base. This is accomplished by taking him off his feet while momentarily balancing him atop your own torso to launch him. For one-arm throws (*ippon seo nage* variations), the arm serves as a lever that produces a longer arc, allowing you to launch him higher and farther, thus increasing his impact with the ground.

Flooring an Assailant

You can put an assailant on the ground in three ways:

1. *Undermine his balance.* Combatives include strikes, throwing.

2. *Undermine his support.* Combatives include strikes, trips, and leg sweeps, especially on the lead leg as he moves forward and shifts his weight.

3. *Lock his joints to force him down.* When the defender is still standing, a heel hook is especially effective. The heel hook is best applied by using your hip and core, not just your leg. As you move your hip, drag your leg with you to ensnare his leg, while knocking his torso off balance.

Keep in mind that a defender often falls to the ground with an assailant because the assailant grabs or locks on to him while falling. Flailing and grabbing are natural instincts when falling to the ground. Floor an assailant both strategically and tactically to attack his vulnerabilities—eyes, throat, and groin.

To control an adversary's center of gravity, a push or pull move is usually used. This type of combative is best used when perpendicular to the adversary's center of gravity, when neither of his legs can easily recover to restore his balance. The goal is to remove both his support and balance simultaneously. Takedowns, sweeps, and throws displace an opponent's foot or shift his center of mass away from a remaining support leg(s).

The formula is once again simple: krav maga is designed to overcome any disparities in size or strength. The key is *simultaneous attack and defense* to disrupt the attack. As soon as you disrupt the attack, you will immediately redirect it into a throw or takedown, using gravity and the ground to further neutralize the threat. A strong combative will stun the assailant, allowing you to enter and unbalance him so you can complete the takedown or throw.

An unbalanced adversary is obviously easier to displace than a balanced one. Even if your initial throw or takedown is unsuccessful and the assailant maintains partial balance, continue your retzev, applying a subsequent combative or series of combatives to keep attacking the threat. Always attempt to keep your retzev seamless, transitioning from one technique to another in a logical manner.

When an assailant attempts to throw you, by the very nature of movement and tactics, he is creating an opening for you to counterthrow. This is true of all combatives, including kicks, punches, knees, and elbows. A good fighter will minimize these openings, but they are still there to be exploited if the defender is skilled enough to recognize and execute the countertechnique properly.

The following throws and takedowns are designed for both civilians and professionals who may be wearing law enforcement and military tactical gear. These tactics are specifically designed to help diminish the likelihood that the kravist will become entangled with the assailant. In addition, these techniques account for the extra weight load or displacement and mobility restriction that professional tactical gear places on the kravist. *Each of the following throws assumes the defender is on the assailant's right side and has just defended a right straight punch.* Included are the Japanese names for these takedowns and throws, as these are transliterated in the Israeli krav maga curriculum.

Outside Reverse Sweep (Osoto Gari)

For the outside reverse sweep, or *osoto gari*, you'll take out an opponent's legs by sweeping your outside leg against and into his inside knee or lower leg(s). For maximum effect you can combine the sweep with a strike, shove, or hook to the neck. You can target one or both of the opponent's legs and knees.

Stand with your right side to your opponent's left side. Straighten and strengthen your right leg to sweep your opponent's left leg. Grab your opponent's right wrist with your left hand, and place your right hand firmly on his shoulder. Push your opponent diagonally toward a ten o'clock position with your hands, as you bring your heel back and up against his knee or leg in a chopping motion. Jolt your opponent forward while simultaneously sweeping back. This technique will take your opponent's upper body forward and his lower body back. You must time this move exquisitely to sweep your opponent before he can counter the move to sweep you first. After your opponent goes down, follow up with kicks and stomps to the head, neck, solar plexus, ribs, groin, fingers, and other targets of opportunity.

Note: You can also hook your same-side arm around your opponent and use it to pull him in toward you as you sweep backward through his nearside leg.

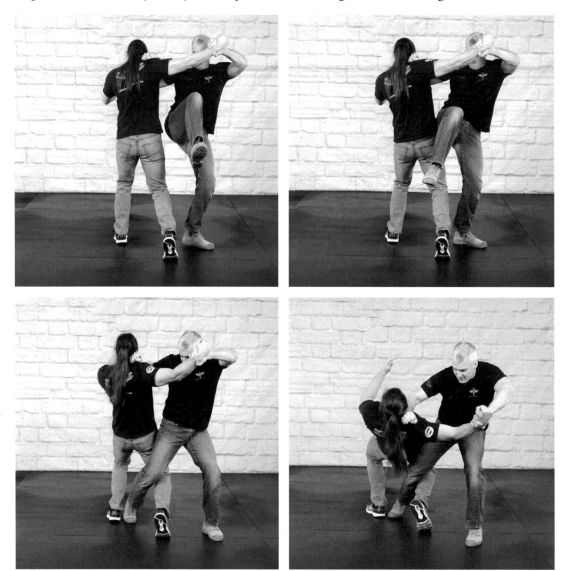

Outside reverse sweep (osoto gari).

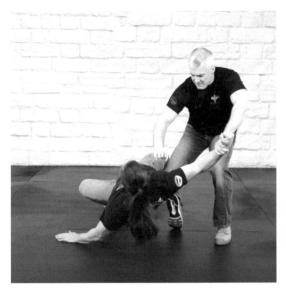 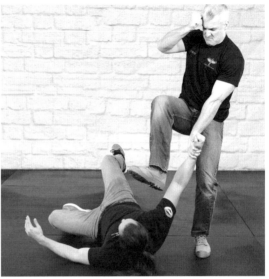

Outside reverse sweep (osoto gari).

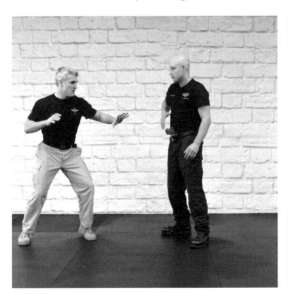 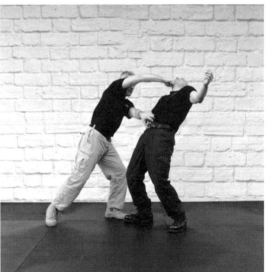

Outside reverse sweep (osoto gari) to remove a handgun from an assailant's waistband.

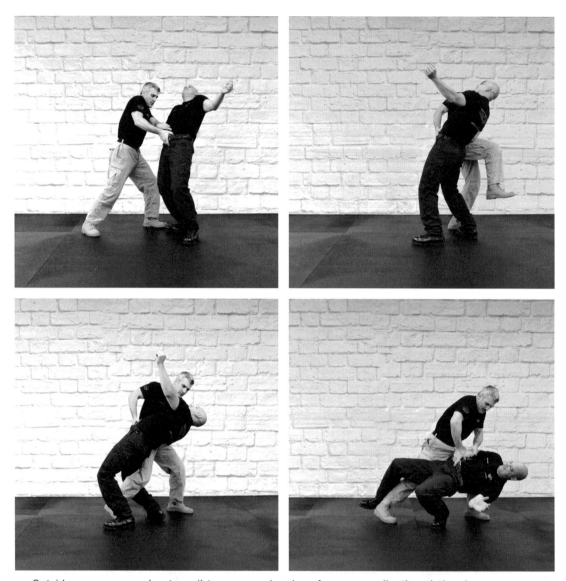

Outside reverse sweep (osoto gari) to remove a handgun from an assailant's waistband.

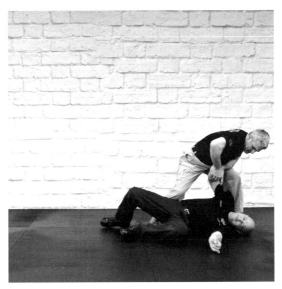

Outside reverse sweep (osoto gari) to remove a handgun from an assailant's waistband.

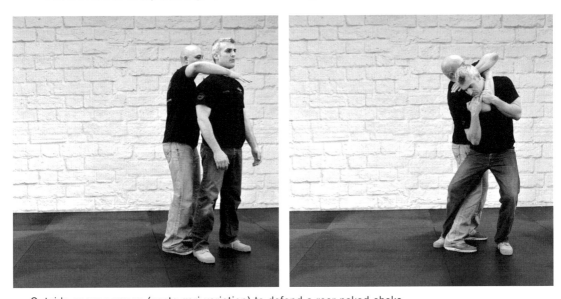

Outside reverse sweep (osoto gari variation) to defend a rear naked choke.

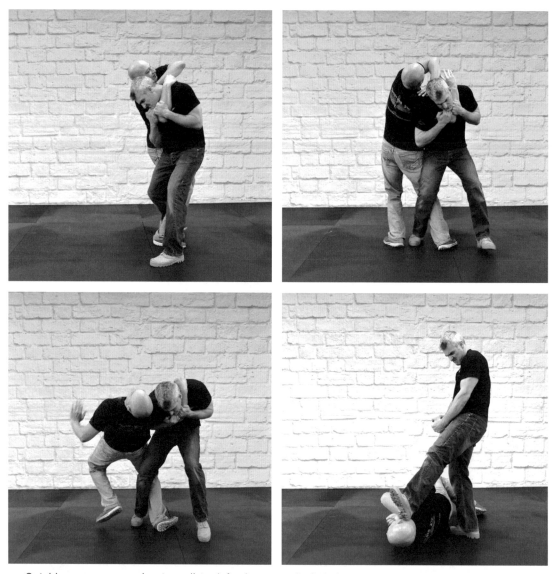

Outside reverse sweep (osoto gari) to defend a rear naked choke.

Rear Tackle Trip (Kosoto Gake)

When you are unarmed and have no choice but to attempt to disarm a third party threatening others, or in an active-shooter situation, it is best to use a gross motor movement to surprise the gunman from the rear. A rear tackle trip, or *kosoto gake*, variation works well against a stationary or moving gunman. The tackle is one of the most effective takedown techniques. Like other combatives, the tackle's power derives from hip and leg explosion. Focus on driving your shoulder just below your adversary's hips or midsection with your head to one side of his torso. Bull your neck and keep your face up. Just prior to contact, sink your hips with a wide leg base to explode through your adversary. This is similar to rising from a weight-lifting squat or dead lift, but you will also churn your legs for momentum.

Wrap your arms around the gunman's waist or hips to drive him forward. Our natural reaction when being driven forward is to put our hands out in front to deal with the impact of falling face first, so he may drop the weapon, either a handgun or long gun. (The tactic is the same for a handgun or long gun.) Secure him tightly on the way down, keeping your head buried, prepared to let go just as the gunman collides with the ground. If the gunman does not release the handgun, you must again quickly take his back, while pounding him with one arm and securing the weapon with a good portion of your weight on it. If he continues to hold the handgun, secure the barrel with your right arm to wrench it from his grip. With a firm grip, rotate the handgun's barrel down and away and use it as a cold weapon (an impact weapon). Get up, create distance, and place the weapon back in battery.

Active-Shooter Takedown if the Gunman Releases the Handgun

If the gunman releases the weapon as he is driven into the ground, continue to take his back, administering strong combatives to his head and neck, using forearms, elbows, punches, or palm-heel strikes, perhaps followed by a stomp, as you get up quickly after neutralizing him. (Note: When disarming a long gun, you may be able to choke him with the weapon. But, in the event of a handgun disarm, beware of choking him if he maintains possession, as he can simply shoot you in the head when you attempt to choke him.) Secure and use the handgun as necessary in a cold-weapon capacity.

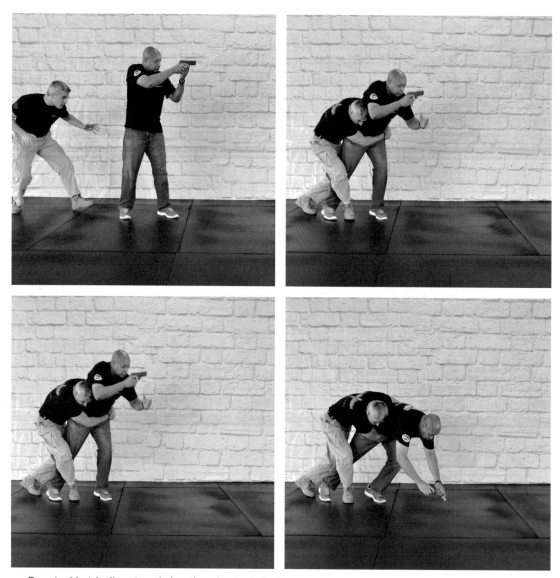

Rear tackle trip (kosoto gake) active-shooter takedown.

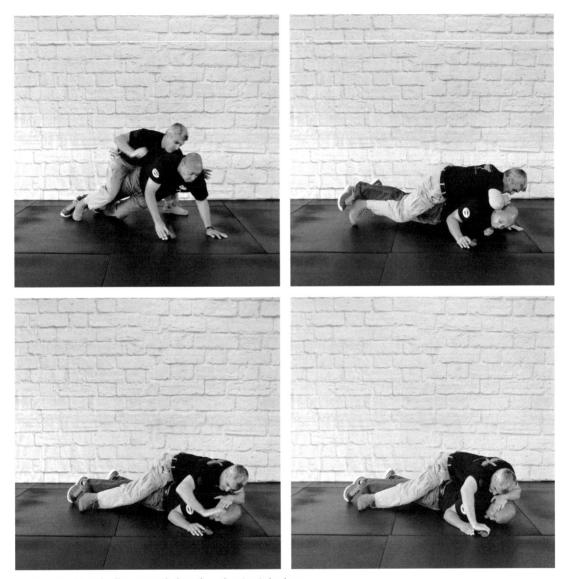

Rear tackle trip (kosoto gake) active-shooter takedown.

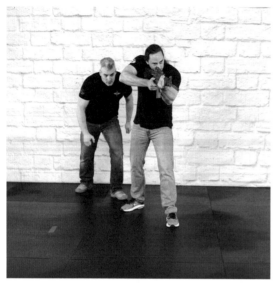 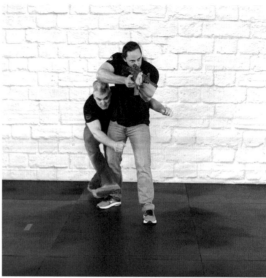

Rear tackle trip (kosoto gake) active-shooter takedown, front view.

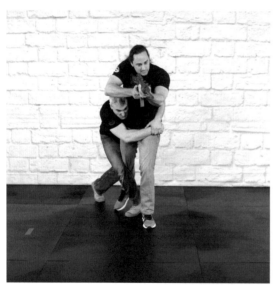 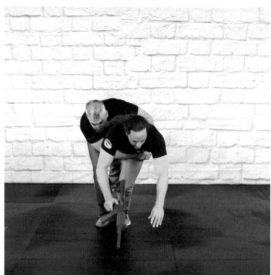

Rear tackle trip active-shooter takedown, front view.

Cavalier #1 Wristlock Takedown

The cavalier #1 wristlock is designed to use your powerful hip-muscle groups and body weight to torque an opponent's wrist to take him down—also establishing strong control over a weapon for removal, if the opponent is holding one. A cavalier #1 is usually preceded by retzev combatives against the assailant, including full-force strikes to the groin, neck, eyes, and other vulnerable targets of opportunity. Properly executed, cavalier #1 would force an opponent to travel three times as far and three times as fast as your pivot if he were to remain on his feet. This powerful takedown places enormous pressure on an opponent's wrist, forcing him down to the ground, while enabling strong control of a weapon. If necessary, you can follow up with a strong kick to the head, midsection, or groin, along with an armbar or wristlock to remove a weapon.

After administering combatives, for cavalier #1, secure your opponent's right hand while you are positioned behind his right shoulder and to his side. If you are securing your opponent's right hand for the takedown, place your right hand on top of his right hand or "knuckles to knuckles." Your left hand then secures his right forearm just above the wrist. Do not grab the opponent's wrist, as this will hinder your desired objective of applying maximum torqueing pressure to the wrist. Try to keep your elbows as close to your body as possible to best control the weapon and keep it away from you and directed toward the assailant.

The wrist is flexible, but few people are flexible if you apply simultaneous pressure inward and sideways. Think of the cavalier as driving your opponent's index finger toward his same-side shoulder. To apply the torqueing pressure, as illustrated, take a 180-degree circular, sweeping rear step (tai sabaki) with your left leg. *Do not release the opponent's hand as he falls.* If the opponent continues to present a threat once he is on the ground, you may use a heel stomp to his head or body, depending on your perception of his continued ability to resist. Continue to pull up on his arm, applying pressure to keep his right shoulder off the ground.

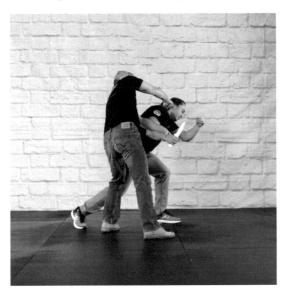 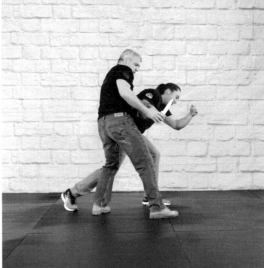

Cavalier #1 wristlock takedown to confiscate an edged weapon.

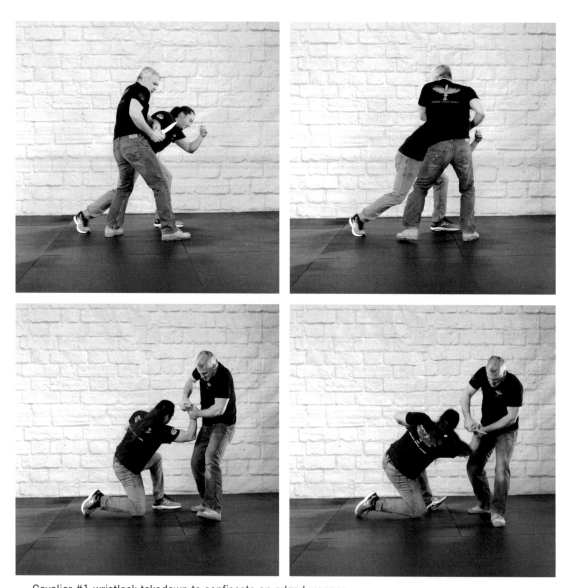

Cavalier #1 wristlock takedown to confiscate an edged weapon.

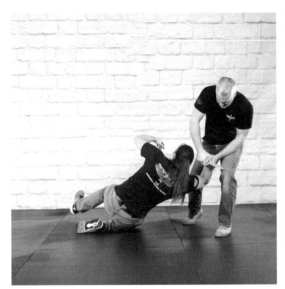 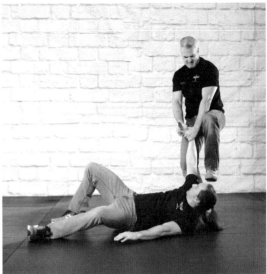

Cavalier #1 wristlock takedown to confiscate an edged weapon.

Note: A common mistake when controlling an edged weapon for the takedown is when the defender brings an opponent's edged weapon across his own throat while applying the cavalier #1 to remove the weapon from the assailant's grip. When you encounter a strong opponent, you may have to continue to "loosen him up." Debilitating him prior to the takedown may require a knee strike, shin kick, or other combative, including a vertical uppercut elbow to the back of his clenched fist. These strikes both distract and physically undermine your adversary's ability to resist.

Your adversary may try to counter the technique by rolling out of the hold using his momentum. Once you have taken your 180-degree, circular, sweeping rear step to take him off his feet, you can prevent his rolling by torqueing his wrist in the opposite direction and pinning it to your thigh. Again, at this point many offensive combatives can be used, such as a heel stomp to the head, midsection, or groin—or, in an unarmed scenario, a scissors armbar that will break the arm.

For law enforcement and security personnel, once you have taken the opponent down on his back, you may reverse him onto his stomach by yanking up on his arm and stepping 180 degrees in the opposite direction, while clipping his arm just below the elbow with your knee, to facilitate his turn. You are then in a strong position to collapse his straight arm for facedown control of the weapon and the application of restraints. An advanced variation utilizes a jumping scissors kick (not depicted) to the opponent's groin, while applying crushing wrist pressure.

Two-Leg Front Tackle Takedown (*Morote Gari*)

The two-leg front tackle takedown, or *morote gari*, is a strong combative that lands an opponent squarely on the back of his head or at least on his back. This example shows this combative executed against a lead straight punch. Depending on your timing, you can parry the straight punch and then slip under it to initiate the takedown or simply slip underneath the punch for the takedown. Bull your neck while keeping your head up as much as possible to see the opponent. Tuck your chin and ram your shoulder through the opponent's midsection or hips. As you make impact using your shoulder, simultaneously wrap both your arms around the crooks of the opponent's knees to take his legs out, aided by a sharp pulling motion. While you can go down with the opponent, optimally, you can remain standing and simply dump the opponent down on his back. A heel stomp to the groin may be immediately available to further incapacitate the opponent.

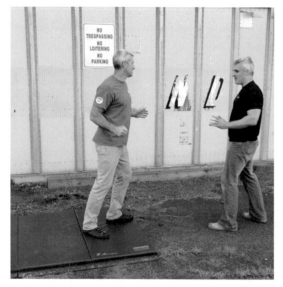 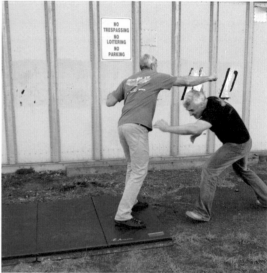

Two-leg front tackle takedown (morote gari) used in defending a straight punch. Be sure to keep your head tight to his hip so he cannot attempt a guillotine counter on his way down.

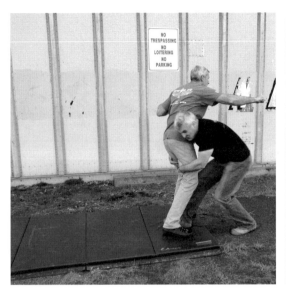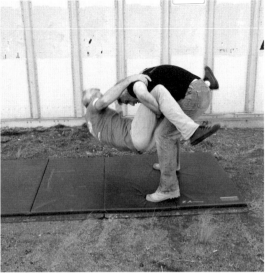

Two-leg front tackle takedown (morote gari) used in defending a straight punch. Note: The defender remains standing. It is also possible to pancake the opponent, but this would place the defender on the ground—a less desirable result. Always try to remain standing.

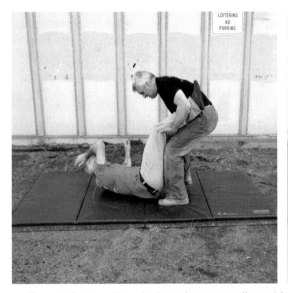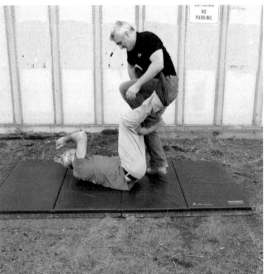

Two-leg front tackle takedown (morote gari) used in defending a straight punch.

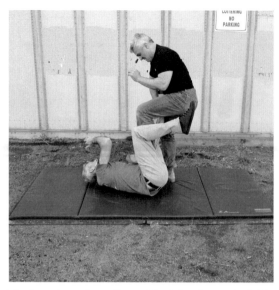

Two-leg front tackle takedown (morote gari) used in defending a straight punch.

Bucket Takedown (Te Guruma)

The bucket takedown, or *te guruma*, is a potent takedown that allows you to strike the opponent's groin from the rear while dropping him facedown onto the ground. This technique can be used as a follow-up to many techniques, including an outside block against a hook or the sliding punch defense. While not depicted, this technique may also be used as a frontal combative to slam an opponent to the ground with your body weight on top of him.

The bucket takedown takes you to your opponent's deadside, optimally pinning his closest arm to you with your left arm and shoulder while slamming your right forearm between his legs. As you strike or grab his testicles, position your hips slightly behind him to launch him forward or "dump" him to the ground face first. It is also possible to pick the opponent up and turn him 180 degrees to slam his head into the ground. Pinning his arm will hinder his ability to cushion his fall. Sink your hips into your opponent, and keep your back straight. As with all takedowns, power emanates from your hips and core. Explode up, keeping your back straight and head tucked, to avoid an elbow counterstrike from his free arm. The forward throwing motion loosely resembles pouring out a bucket, hence the name.

The specific defense depicted allows you to deflect an incoming rear punch or cross, while simultaneously moving away from the punch and delivering your own straight punch counterattack to the throat, chin, nose, midsection, or groin.

To defend against the incoming straight punch, the key is to deflect and step off the line, moving both feet together. Do not lunge; keep your feet equidistant by moving them the same distance. You may also punch low to the assailant's body, targeting his liver, or deliver a hand strike to his groin. (These last two counterstrikes are useful against assailants whose height advantage does not allow you to easily reach their head to counterattack.)

From your left outlet stance, step to your left while bringing your left cupped hand diagonally across your face, close to your right shoulder. Your hand will lead your body defense to redirect the adversary's punch by sliding down your adversary's right arm while your right arm delivers a half-roundhouse counterpunch to the throat, chin, or nose. After you close the distance on your assailant with your simultaneous counterpunch, to execute the bucket takedown, transition your punching arm to control his torso. As you transition into the throw, sink your hips and thrust your other arm through the assailant's legs to first strike and then grab his groin. Load your hips properly by bending your knees with your back straight. Forcefully clutch the assailant's testicles to lift him up and forward to—in krav maga parlance—"bucket dump" him facedown or on his head. Once you dump him face first, continue with any additional combatives—such as heel stomps or taking his back—while administering punches or elbows to the back of his head or neck.

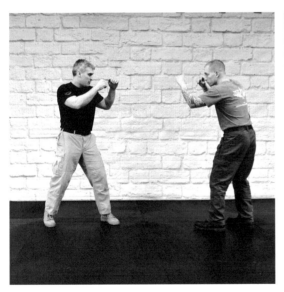 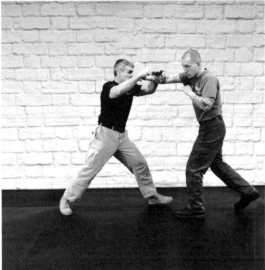

Bucket takedown (te guruma) used in defending a straight punch.

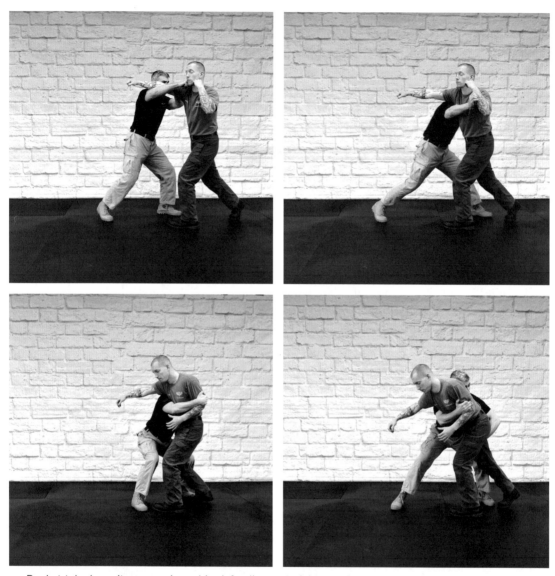

Bucket takedown (te guruma) used in defending a straight punch.

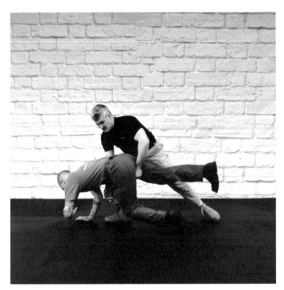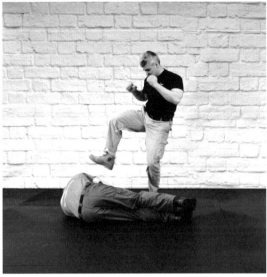

Bucket takedown (te guruma) used in defending a straight punch.

Krav Maga Throws

Defending a Hook Punch into Throws

Imi incorporated the following throws (using the transliterated Japanese names) into the Israeli krav maga curriculum. These techniques may be used after initially defending a hook punch. (The same throwing principles apply as covered in the previous straight-punch sliding defenses.)

- Koshi guruma
- Ogoshi
- Ippon seoi nage

Hook-Punch Defense into Neck Throw (Koshi Guruma)

The 360 outside punch defense combined with stepping off the line of attack to the outside facilitates the neck throw, or *koshi guruma* (hip wheel throw). I call this a neck throw because the defender is securing the opponent by his neck. After initially blocking the punch, while stepping offline to stun the assailant, you can apply the koshi guruma neck throw by using the correct footwork and turning your torso into the assailant. Do not begin the throwing action until you have the assailant off balance by forcing his weight decidedly forward over his feet.

Defend from your left outlet stance. Step off the line while blocking and counterattacking. After stunning the assailant, step diagonally with your right foot to the inside of the assailant's (right) foot. As you perform a crossover step, begin angling your body, and slide the left heel to the inside of the assailant's (left) nearside foot. These two entry steps turn your back into the assailant's torso. Your (right) hip must be positioned outside of the assailant's (right) hip. Pull the assailant's right arm straight out and around you to unbalance him to his right front while your right arm around the back of his neck simultaneously pulls him forward toward you, creating a whipsaw effect. Your bodies must be glued together with no slack.

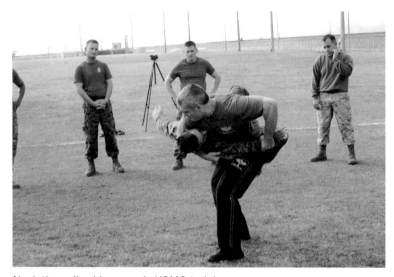

Neck throw (koshi guruma), USMC training.

As you shift onto the ball of your left foot, simultaneously pull forward quickly with your left arm into a circular motion. To throw the assailant, bend your knees to obtain leverage, with your hips below the assailant's hips. As you pull the assailant forward, shift your weight onto the balls of your feet, slightly flexing your knees for balance. Be sure to tightly control his lower neck and upper shoulders. Essentially, you are delivering an arimi, or slightly bent forearm strike, to the back of his neck or upper shoulders, depending on what kind of grip you have on him. You will be able to whipsaw him as you yank forward with his arm and jettison him over your hips. Squeeze tightly, straighten your legs, and rotate your torso by pulling forward in a decisive circular motion. This allows you to rotate him over your right hip to upend and smash him into the ground. Finish with a heel kick if necessary.

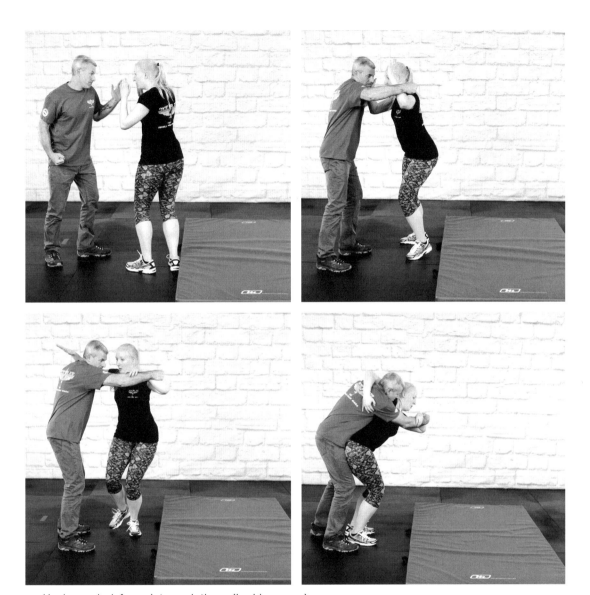

Hook-punch defense into neck throw (koshi guruma).

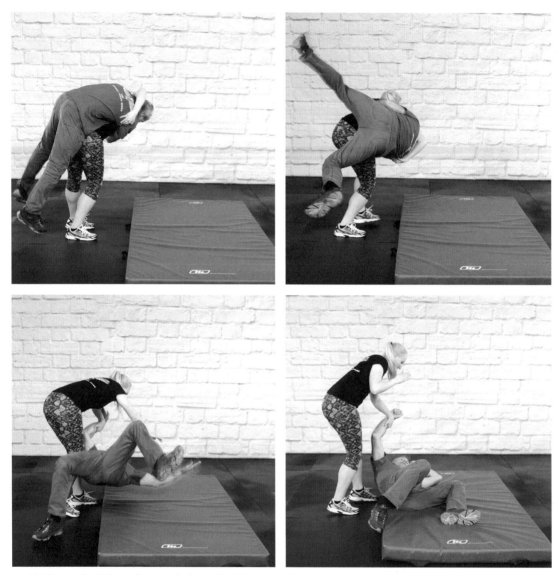

Hook-punch defense into neck throw (koshi guruma).

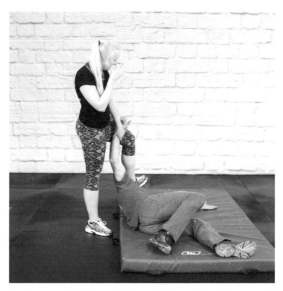

Hook-punch defense into neck throw (koshi guruma).

Hook Punch Defense into Hip Throw (Ogoshi)

The 360 outside-punch defense combined with stepping off the line of attack to the outside facilitates the hip throw, or *ogoshi*. After initially blocking the punch, while stepping offline to stun the assailant, you can apply the hip throw by using the correct footwork and turning your torso into the assailant. Do not begin the throwing action until you have the assailant off balance by forcing his weight decidedly forward over his feet.

Defend from your left outlet stance. Step off the line while blocking and counterattacking. After stunning the assailant, step diagonally with your right foot to the inside of the assailant's (right) foot. As you perform a crossover step, begin angling your body, and slide the left heel to the inside of the assailant's (left) nearside foot. These two entry steps turn your back into the assailant's torso. Your right hip must be positioned outside of the assailant's right hip. Pull the assailant's right arm straight out and around you to unbalance him to his right front. Your right arm around his torso simultaneously pulls him forward toward you, creating a whipsaw effect. Your bodies must be glued together with no slack.

As you shift onto the ball of your left foot, simultaneously pull with your left arm forward quickly into a circular motion. To throw the assailant, bend your knees to obtain leverage, with your hips below the assailant's hips. As you pull the assailant forward, shift your weight onto the balls of your feet, slightly flexing your knees for balance. Be sure to tightly control his upper body. Squeeze tightly, straighten your legs, and rotate your torso by pulling forward in a decisive circular motion. This allows you to rotate him over your right hip, upending him and smashing him into the ground. Finish with a heel kick if necessary.

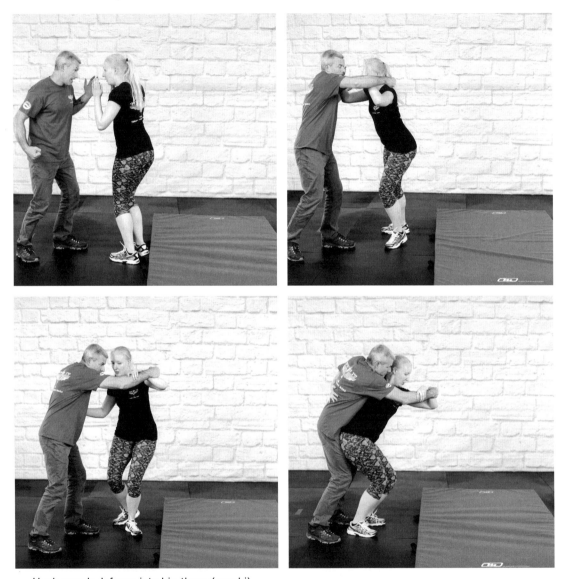

Hook-punch defense into hip throw (ogoshi).

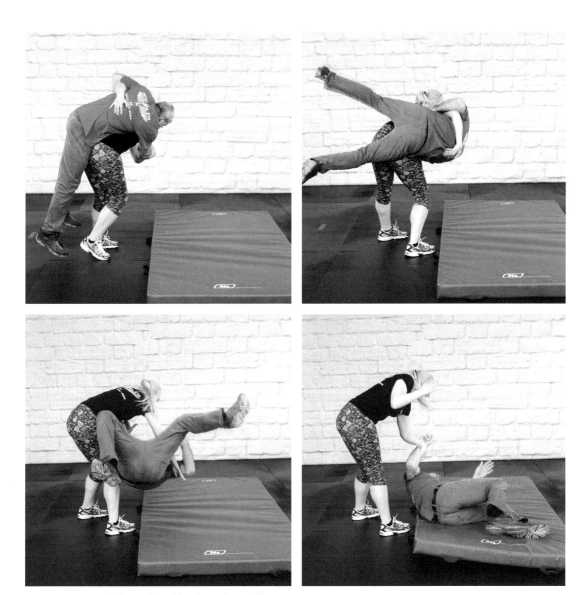

Hook-punch defense into hip throw (ogoshi).

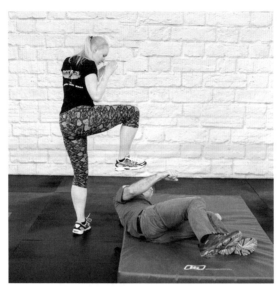

Hook-punch defense into hip throw (ogoshi).

Straight-Punch Defense into the One-Arm Break and Throw (Ippon Seoi Nage)

The one-arm break and throw, or *ippon seoi nage*, is a throw tailor made for this particular krav maga defense. After initially blocking or parrying the punch, depending on the attack, you must quickly secure the assailant's punching arm. Naturally, he will retract the arm. Therefore, your over-the-top punch must stun him, allowing you to isolate his arm. While stepping off the line, simultaneously counterpunch and secure his arm with your free (rear) arm. Using the correct footwork, while turning your torso into the assailant with proper body positioning, apply the one-arm break and throw.

From your left outlet stance, sidestep his incoming punch while delivering a sliding over-the-top counterpunch defense. Keep your thumb pointed up, allowing your inverted punch to drive his arm down while sliding your own arm atop of his to deliver the punch. Stun the attacker because, otherwise, he will naturally retract his arm, thereby thwarting the throw attempt. After you deliver the stunning blow to the assailant's head, secure the assailant's right arm, and step forward with your left leg. This will turn your body 90 degrees to initiate the throw.

As you perform a crossover step with your right foot to switch your stance and complete the angling of your body, simultaneously snake your left counterattack arm underneath the assailant's right arm above his elbow joint. This fits the *V* of your bent elbow snugly into his armpit. The trapezius and deltoids of your right side should be directly inside the assailant's arm with your left side extremely close to his front. Keep the assailant's right arm secured with your left hand at his wrist. If you wish to break the assailant's arm, secure his arm with his palm facing up to create an armbar that turns into an arm break. As you launch him, yank both your hands down and to your right to throw the assailant over your right shoulder. Bend your knees, positioning yourself with your hips in line with his groin or as low as possible and keeping your upper body straight to lift the assailant onto your back.

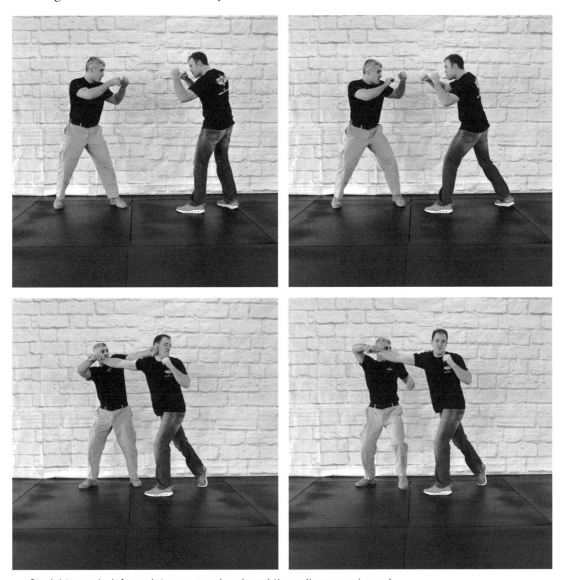

Straight-punch defense into one-arm break and throw (ippon seoi nage).

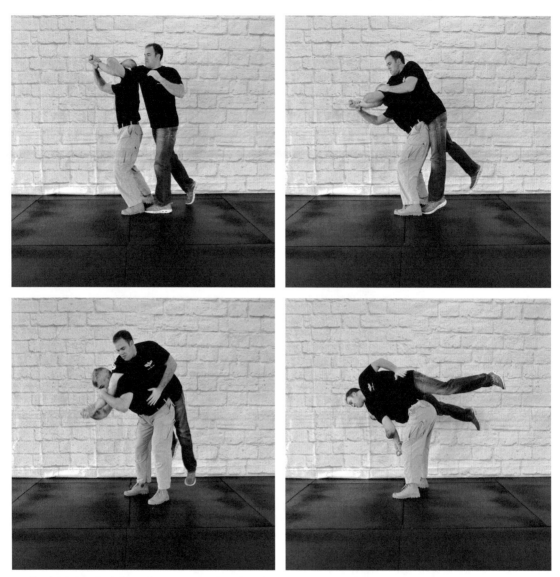

Straight-punch defense into one-arm break and throw (ippon seoi nage).

Arm Throw (Ippon Seoi Nage) Variation

A variation of ippon seoi nage is to drop to one or both knees to hurl the assailant over your shoulder. Because you are closer to the ground (having dropped to your knees), the impact on the assailant may be less; nevertheless, this is an effective method. The knee-drop variation may be used when a defender initially struggles or is forced forward. In the sequence below, the defender drops to both her knees to maximize the whipsaw throwing effect.

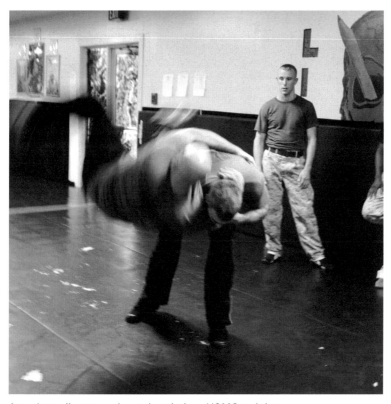

Arm throw (ippon seoi nage) variation, USMC training.

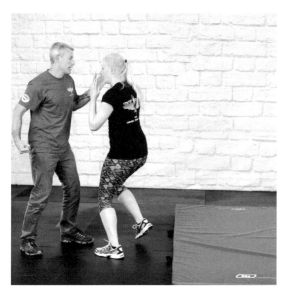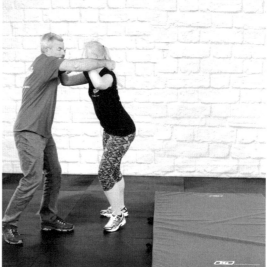

Hook-punch defense into arm throw (ippon seoi nage) variation.

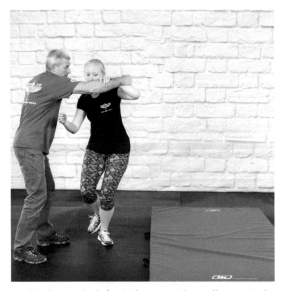
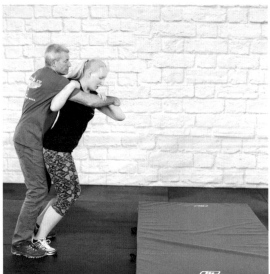

Hook-punch defense into arm throw (ippon seoi nage) variation.

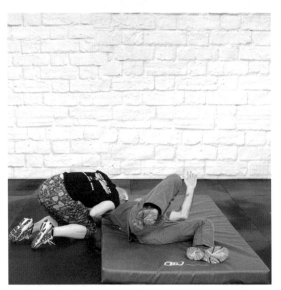
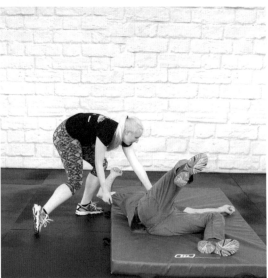

Hook-punch defense into arm throw (ippon seoi nage) variation.

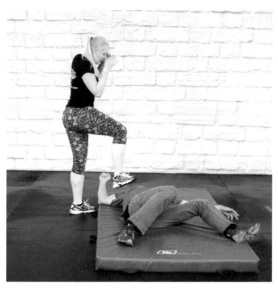

Hook-punch defense into arm throw (ippon seoi nage) variation.

Scissors Legs Sweep (Kani Basame)

Should you find yourself in the undesirable position of being on the ground with a standing opponent trying to gain position on you, the scissors legs sweep, or *kani basame*, is a formidable takedown option. The goal is to take the opponent facedown and take his back to deliver debilitating blows. With correct timing, when on your side, use your bottom leg to catch and trap the opponent's nearside leg in the vicinity of his ankle. Simultaneously, with your top leg, deliver a strong modified roundhouse kick for a forward kani basame—or a reverse roundhouse kick for a reverse kani basame—to the opponent's knee crook. The combined lower-leg trap and upper-leg roundhouse-type kick buckle the opponent's knee, taking him facedown. As the opponent goes down, immediately transition to taking his back. Deliver follow-on combatives such as the horizontal #1 elbow strikes depicted or any other debilitating combatives. Get up. If necessary, deliver additional heel kicks to incapacitate the opponent.

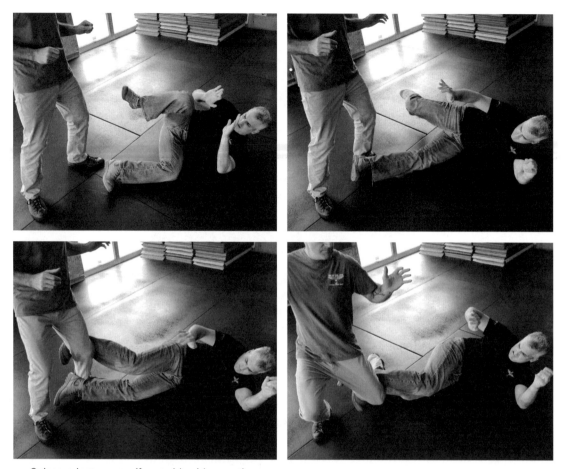

Scissors legs sweep (forward kani basame).

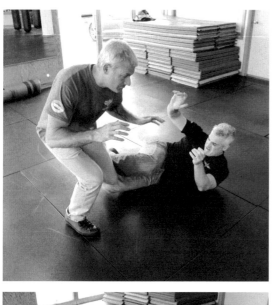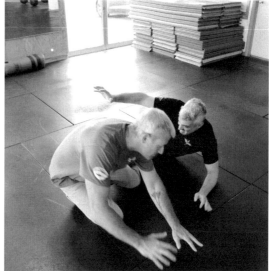

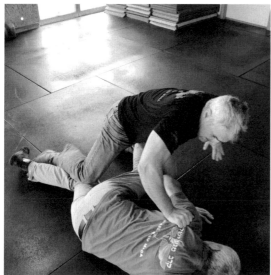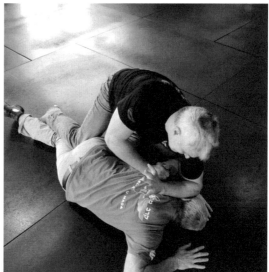

Scissors legs sweep (forward kani basame).

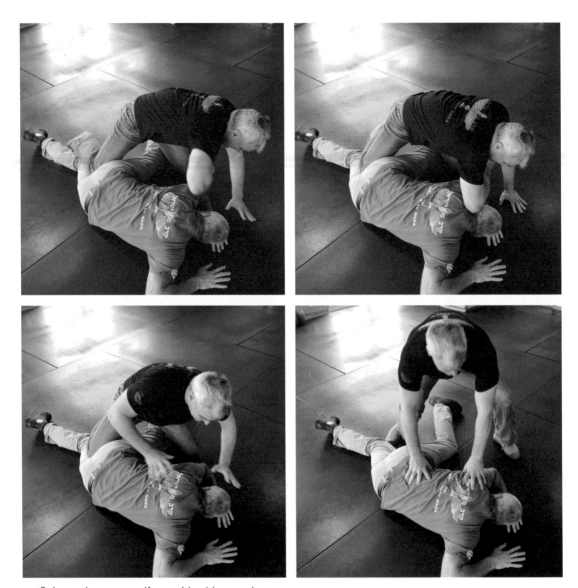

Scissors legs sweep (forward kani basame).

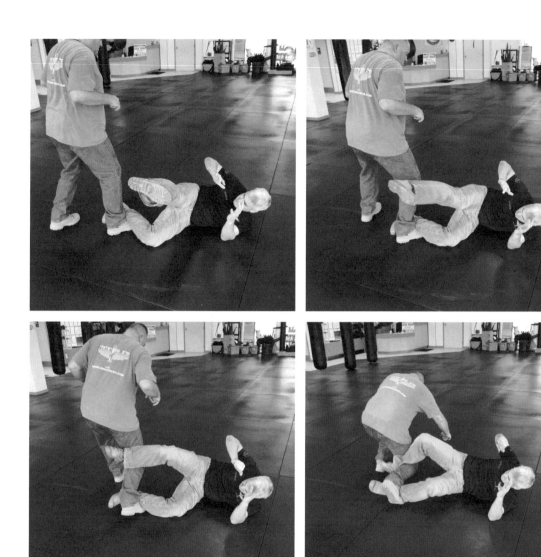

Scissors legs sweep (reverse kani basame).

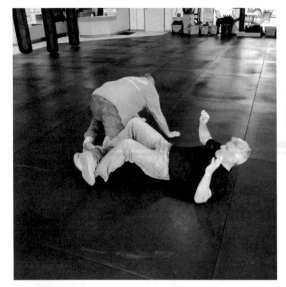
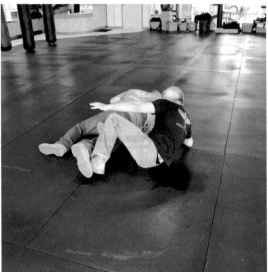
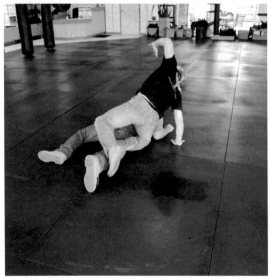
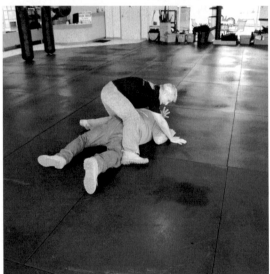

Scissors legs sweep (reverse kani basame).

Note: The scissors legs sweep may also be performed when the defender is facing away from the attacker, should the attacker attempt to go around the defender to reach the defender's back. In this case, the defender reverses scissors movement to deliver a heel kick to the back of the attacker's knee crook while trapping the front of the attacker's ankle and foot. Obviously, it is better for the defender not to present his back to the attacker, either while standing or on the ground. Accordingly, there is a de-emphasis on the reverse scissors legs sweep with the defender's back to the attacker.

Side Kick Leg-Trap Takedown

Should you find yourself in the undesirable position of being on the ground with a standing opponent trying to gain position on you, the side kick leg trap is another formidable takedown option. The goal is to take the opponent down on his back by damaging his knee with a modified foot trap and side kick. With correct timing, when on your side, use your bottom leg to catch and trap the opponent's nearside leg in the vicinity of his Achilles. Simultaneously, use your top leg to deliver a strong modified side kick to the opponent's vulnerable knee. Combining your lower leg trap and upper leg side kick will buckle the opponent's knee, taking him on his back. As the opponent goes down, immediately get up to deliver additional heel kicks to incapacitate him.

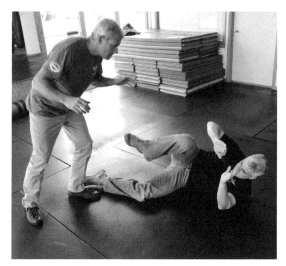
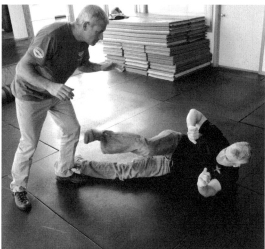
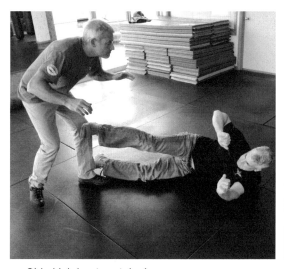
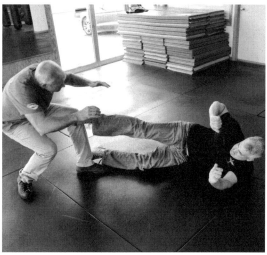

Side kick leg-trap takedown.

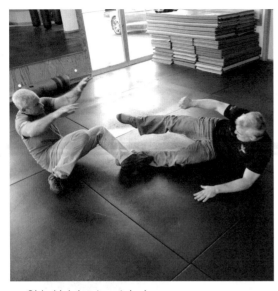 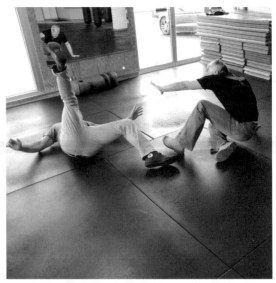

Side kick leg-trap takedown.

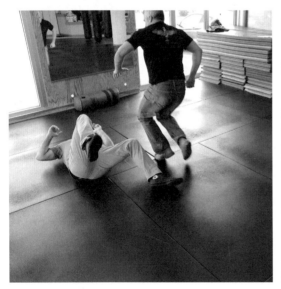 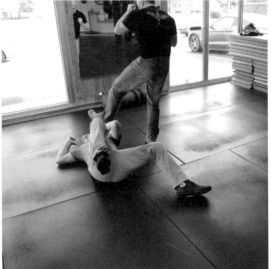

Side kick leg-trap takedown.

CHAPTER 7

Armbars, Finger Manipulations, Leg Locks, and Leg Triangle Chokes

---

Combatives Family #12: Armbars, Finger Manipulations, Leg Locks, and Leg Triangle Chokes

---

Armbars

For ground survival, Israeli krav maga uses a few simple armbars that enable a kravist to dislocate an opponent's elbow—or worse. To damage or break a joint, you simply force the joint in a direction it is not evolutionarily designed to go. Joints move in six basic directions: extension, flexion, supination, pronation, adduction, and abduction. To inflict maximum damage with an armbar, place as much distance as possible between the applied force (your grip) and the fulcrum (your inner thigh). The opponent's arm is the lever. The goal is to damage the opponent's elbow ligaments and tendons by forcing the elbow joint to bend beyond its natural anatomical limits. A forcibly applied straight armbar stands a strong chance of dislocating the elbow. In addition, keep your back straight when dropping your back to the floor. This adds your maximum weight to the armbar lever mechanism. Note: As you go to the ground, be sure to tuck your chin so as not to bash your own head into the ground.

Straight Armbar from the Mount

Krav maga uses two straight-armbar variations with a few different leg-placement options to isolate the elbow joint. Straight armbars almost always follow combatives designed either to distract or injure the opponent prior to the armbar—or any other krav maga joint lock being applied. In the first example, from a mount, after administering a strong combative to the opponent's head, secure the opponent's targeted arm with both your arms. Rise to a kneeling position with your far-side leg while keeping the opponent's arm firmly trapped to your torso. When you secure the opponent's arm, you must stretch it to its maximum extension as though you were pulling his arm out of its socket. Once you have risen to your outside knee and secured the targeted arm, swing your inside leg over the opponent's face to prevent his escape or defense. Squeeze both your thighs together as you explosively drop your back to the ground. You must keep your hips and buttocks close to the opponent's torso. The most common mistake is creating separation that allows the arm to slip. Be sure to tuck your head and not hold your tongue between your teeth. The strong force of your dropping back, while trapping his arm between your legs, will severely damage the elbow joint. Take care to angle the opponent's arm across your thigh and not straight across your groin. (Those who train with groin protection often make this mistake. Be assured, if you then do this in a nontraining defensive situation without groin protection, you are in for a painful surprise.) **Be careful in practice not to injure your partner.**

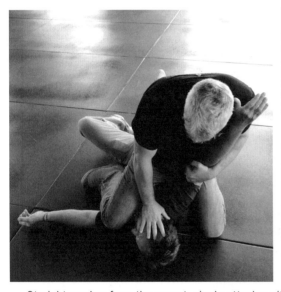 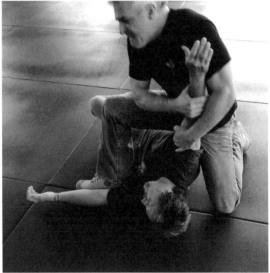

Straight armbar from the mount, single-attacker situation.

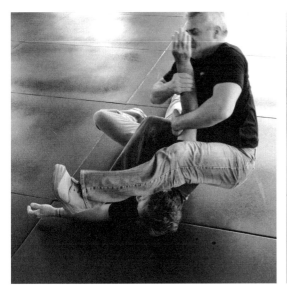
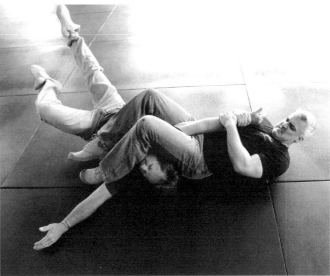

Straight armbar from the mount (single-attacker situation).

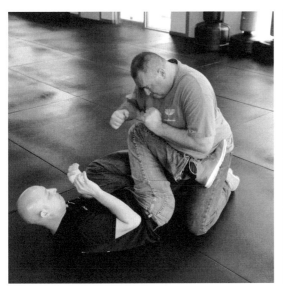
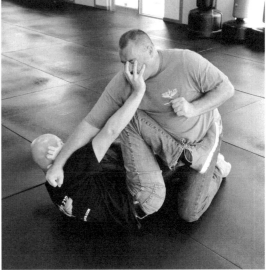

Straight armbar variation in defending a straight punch (single-attacker situation).

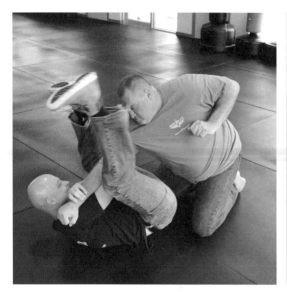 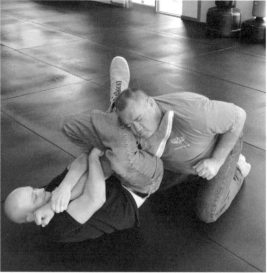

Straight armbar variation in defending a straight punch (single-attacker situation).

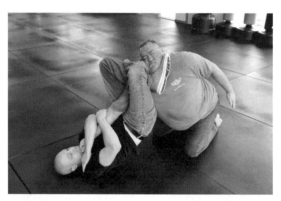

Straight armbar variation in defending a straight punch (single-attacker situation).

Foreleg Brace into Armbar

This is the essential foreleg brace, where the defender turns on one side to prevent the attacker from mounting or pummeling the defender with upper-body attacks. By turning on your side, insert your top foreleg and knee between you and the attacker to keep him or her at bay as you deliver combatives such as eye gouges and throat strikes. The "brakes" technique disengages you from an attacker who is trying to spread your legs or mount you, but it can also serve as a snare to catch and trap the opponent for transitions into straight armbars (and triangle chokes, the next technique presented). Remember: your hips and legs are your most powerful muscles; use them well. The preference is to create separation and damage to the opponent with kicks and then get right to your feet. Again, being on the ground is dangerous for the myriad of reasons previously discussed. Nevertheless, ground survival by necessity incorporates maiming or strangling an opponent.

From the foreleg-brace position, parry the punch by deflecting and sliding up the assailant's right incoming arm with your left arm. Simultaneously attack his eyes with a finger strike, making sure to keep your fingers bent to avoid damaging them. Secure the assailant's outstretched arm by clamping down on it while using your striking hand to secure him at the trapezius, grabbing his shirt to prevent him from retracting his arm. As you clamp down to secure the targeted arm, swing your left leg in front of the assailant's face. Yank back forcefully on his right arm to extend it as much as possible as you extend your left leg across his face. Secure the arm tightly, making sure the elbow joint is above your thighs, and extend your body back as you use your core strength to dislocate the elbow. **Be careful in practice not to injure your partner.**

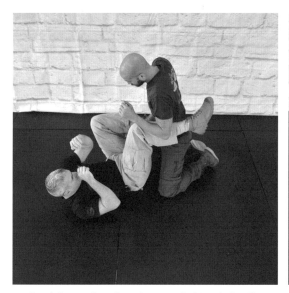 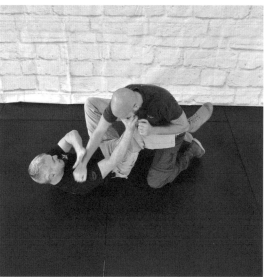

Straight armbar, facedown variation, defending a straight punch (single-attacker situation).

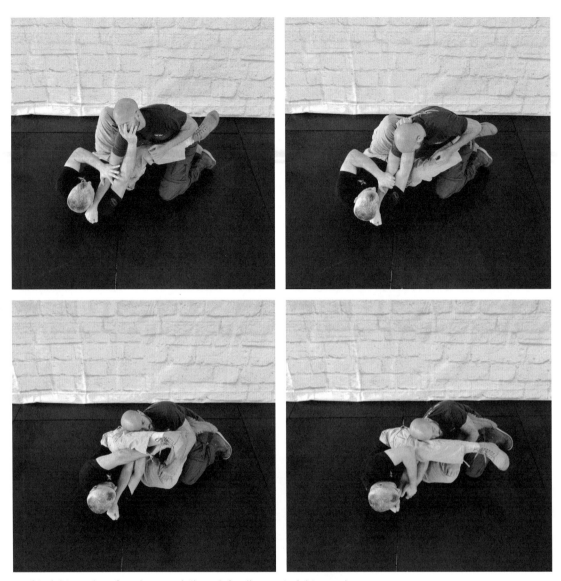

Straight armbar, facedown variation, defending a straight punch.

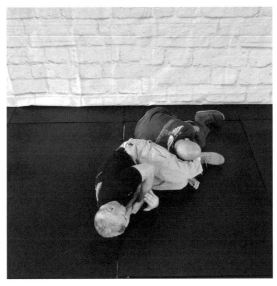

Straight armbar, facedown variation, defending a straight punch.

Finger Manipulations and Breaks

A debilitating tactic to stop an attacker is to break one or more of his fingers. A person is certainly less motivated to fight when part of his hand is broken. Finger manipulations and breaks are easy to learn and apply. As with all joints, the fingers follow a natural articulation. When forced out of their natural articulation, great discomfort ensues. Enough force will disable a finger's movement by dislocation or break. To achieve the best result in finger manipulations and breaks, the finger joint(s) must be isolated.

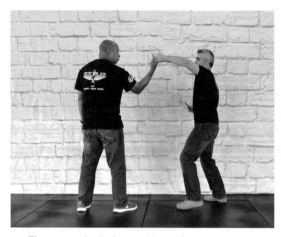

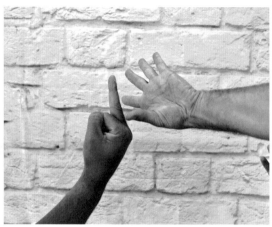

Finger manipulation and breaking.

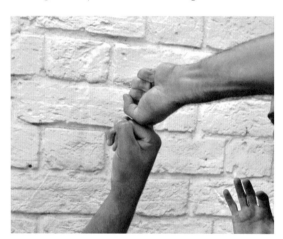

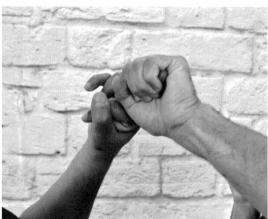

Finger manipulation and breaking.

Leg Locks

As with straight-armbar attacks in a ground-survival situation, Israeli krav maga uses a few simple leg locks that enable a kravist to damage or sever the Achilles tendon, to tear the knee's vital ligaments and tendons, and to dislocate the knee. The leg locks depicted force the tendons and ligaments to stretch beyond their natural range of motion. In addition, certain locks move the knee beyond its natural bend or force it in a direction in which it does not naturally bend. *With all leg locks, be careful not to injure your partner in practice, as the pain receptors from leg locks take longer to reach the brain.* If you do not tap immediately on the first instance of discomfort to indicate your partner is executing the technique correctly, you could be injured.

Achilles Leg Lock

The Achilles leg lock targets the Achilles tendon, hence its name. It can often be applied as a surprise counterattack. The Achilles leg lock is an effective counterattack against an opponent who is trying to pull you into his guard or go to ground with you. It can be applied as a surprise attack as soon as you go to ground with your attacker.

Encircle and trap the opponent's leg with your arm and place the blade of your forearm just above the opponent's ankle, digging it into his Achilles tendon. There are several grip options to secure the opponent's leg. I prefer grabbing my engaged arm with my free arm while placing my nongripping hand against the opponent's shin and placing my foot into his crotch with a heel kick. Do not allow any separation or space between your arm encirclement and his leg. Squeeze the targeted leg tightly with both arms to apply significant pressure to the Achilles. Pincer your legs around your opponent's targeted leg, resting them on his opposite lower thigh to make the lock harder to defend.

Pincer your legs around your opponent's targeted leg, squeezing your knees together to immobilize it. Rest your legs on the lower thigh of his targeted leg to make the lock harder to defend. In addition, you are isolating your targeted stretching pressure because the opponent has no leg movement to alleviate the pressure you apply. After your grip is secure, lean back. This strong body torque, if applied quickly and violently, can rupture or sever the tendon. Note: It is also advantageous to turn the opponent on his side to trap his free leg from kicking you, which he may do anyway in an effort to escape. Trap his free leg against the ground to minimize his ability to kick you with it. You may also deliver heel kicks to the opponent's groin to further incapacitate him.

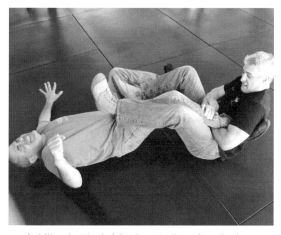 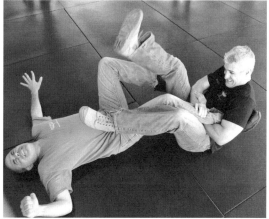

Achilles leg lock (single-attacker situation).

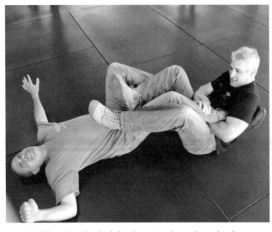 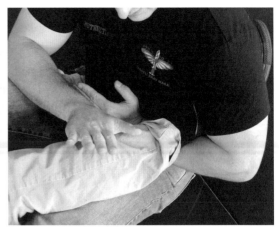

Achilles leg lock (single-attacker situation).

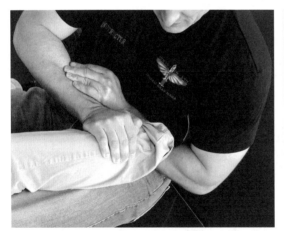 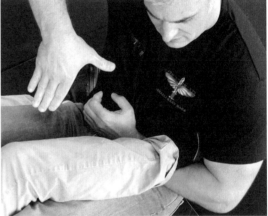

Achilles leg lock, grip option. Note the slight turn in the left arm to drive the radial bone—not the flat of the arm—into the Achilles tendon.

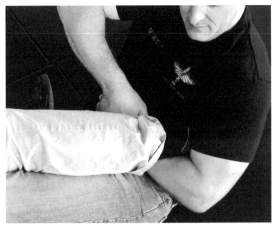

Achilles leg lock, alternative grip option.

Standing Achilles Leg Lock

An Achilles leg lock may also be executed while an opponent is on the ground and you are standing. Place your inside foot against his groin or outer thigh to control his movement. In this case, you want to execute the leg lock against his leg while you are to his outside. Do not attempt the bar while straddling his free leg because he can kick you in the groin. You can also apply the leg lock to an opponent who is standing over you, while you are on the ground, by cinching the Achilles tightly and using your legs to force your opponent off balance or take him down.

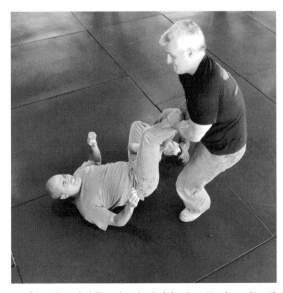
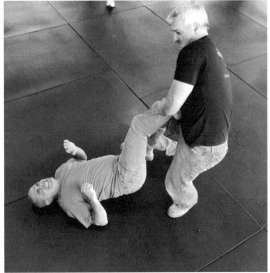

Standing Achilles leg lock (single-attacker situation).

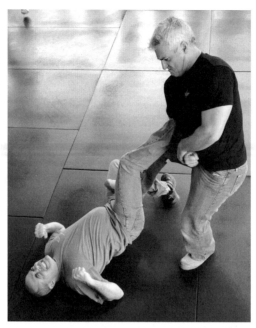

Standing Achilles leg lock, alternative grip option (single-attacker situation).

Ankle-Heel Leg Lock

The ankle-heel leg lock figure-4 is also a highly effective combative to dislocate the ankle and rupture tendons and ligaments. Ankle-heel locks, sometimes known as "toe holds," are often preceded by a takedown. The heel hook is a highly effective technique, attacking the ligaments of the knee in addition to the ankle. Trap the opponent's toes in your armpit while snaking one arm underneath and around his heel. Snake your legs around the opponent's trapped leg and squeeze them together to isolate it and prevent it from moving. By isolating the leg and eliminating any slack in it, you enhance the wrenching, twisting pressure you can apply. Clasp your other arm, and draw the ankle tightly into your body while torqueing to the inside. This ankle-heel lock will place tremendous pressure on the knee ligaments.

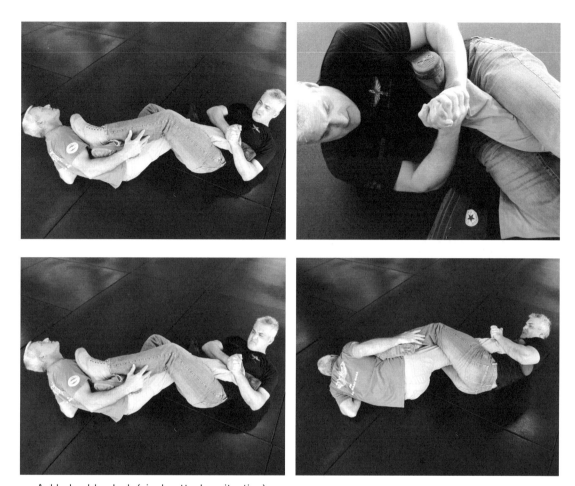

Ankle-heel leg lock (single-attacker situation).

Note: You can easily transition to the inside heel hook from the Achilles leg lock. You will simply release the intended Achilles bar and encircle your arm around the ankle to exert breaking pressure.

Knee-Shredder Lock

Should you find yourself with your back on the ground with an opponent's foot within your grasp near the front of your torso, you can apply a devastating knee-shredder lock. This lock is designed to cause severe damage to the knee by tearing its ligaments. Trap the outside of an opponent's foot (instep facing skyward) and ankle to your chest using both arms. Once again, snake your legs around the opponent's trapped leg to isolate the wrenching, twisting pressure you will apply by eliminating any movement or slack in his leg. Squeeze the leg tightly while wrapping both your legs around the opponent's leg above his knee. If executed properly, the opponent will not be able to wriggle or move his leg. As soon as you have secured the opponent's targeted leg, wrench it sharply, using your body's core strength along with your arms and back. The knee-shredder lock can cause severe damage to the opponent's knee.

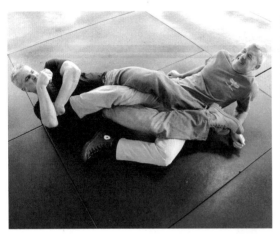 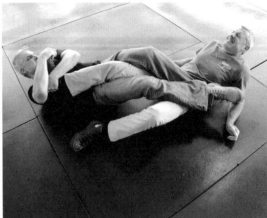

Knee-shredder lock (single-attacker situation).

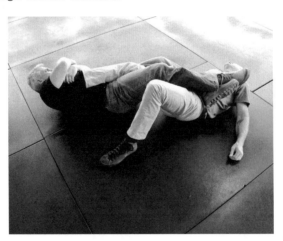

Knee-shredder lock (single-attacker situation).

Knee-Bar Lock

Once again, should you find yourself in the undesirable position of having your back on the ground with a standing opponent's leg near your torso and within your grasp, you can apply a devastating knee-bar lock. The opportunity may come (as depicted) from an opponent attempting to deliver a roundhouse kick or straight heel stomp to your head.

The knee-bar lock is designed to cause damage to the knee by hyperextending or dislocating it. Trap the outside of an opponent's lower leg against your nearside arm. Wrap your lower arm from the inside out around the opponent's leg. Simultaneously secure the opponent's leg with your other arm. As you latch both arms onto the leg, fold both your legs toward the opponent. Use your nearside leg to wrap around the opponent's lower hamstring and knee while simultaneously wrapping your other leg around the opponent's targeted leg. Cross your legs to form a vise, or figure-4 lock, around the opponent's rear leg. Squeeze the opponent's leg tightly with all your limbs. Once you have a boa-constrictor-type hold around the opponent's leg, force him forward. Keep the leg tight to your hip with your torso facing his kneecap. You must not allow his leg to slide forward within your hold. As you force him facedown to the ground, begin to extend or straighten your torso. Your entire body torque and strength is working against his kneecap to damage it.

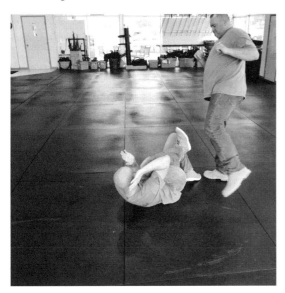 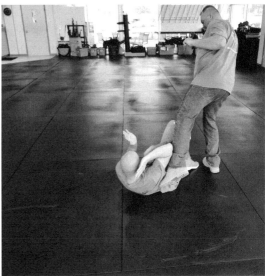

Knee-bar lock defending a roundhouse kick while on the ground (single-attacker situation).

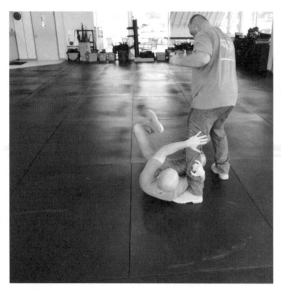
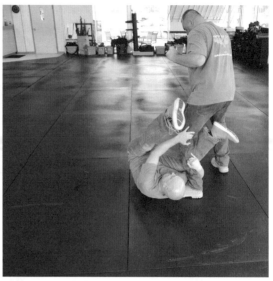

Knee-bar lock defending a roundhouse kick while on the ground (single-attacker situation).

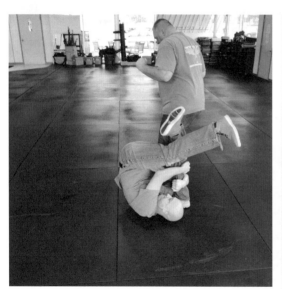
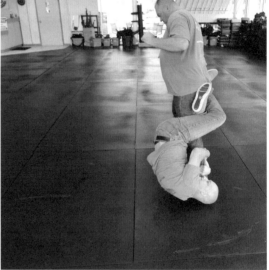

Knee-bar lock defending a roundhouse kick while on the ground (single-attacker situation).

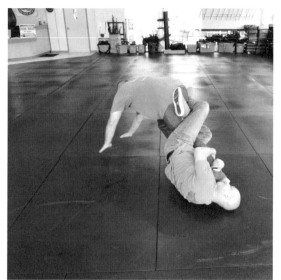
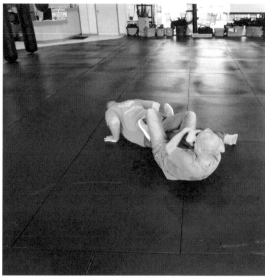

Knee-bar lock defending a roundhouse kick while on the ground (single-attacker situation).

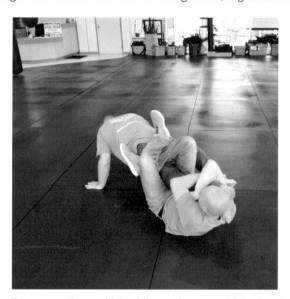

Knee-bar lock defending a roundhouse kick while on the ground (single-attacker situation).

Short Triangle Choke with the Legs

Surviving on the ground sometimes means maiming or strangling the enemy. We can use the arms for this, as previously covered in professional rear naked chokes, and the legs can be used for this as well. As always, any ground combatives that require you to lock up with an opponent will place you in jeopardy of a third party attacking you, especially with stomps to the head.

Foreleg Brace into Short Triangle Choke

The foreleg brace also allows transitions into triangle choke holds. (Again, the best-case scenario is to create space, damage with kicks, and get to your feet.) This example is designed for defenders with shorter legs. From the foreleg brace position, parry the punch by deflecting and sliding up the assailant's right incoming arm with your left arm. Simultaneously attack his eyes with a fingers strike, making sure to keep your fingers bent to avoid damaging them. Secure the assailant's outstretched arm by forcefully clamping down on it while swinging your right leg over his left shoulder. As you clamp down on his head and shoulders, raise your left leg up slightly to insert your right ankle in the crook of your left knee, creating the short triangle choke. This restricts blood flow on both sides of his neck. Squeeze your right leg down into his head while simultaneously clamping down on your right leg with your left leg to optimize the human vice. Pull his head toward you with your right arm to further increase the choking pressure. **Be careful in training not to injure your partner.**

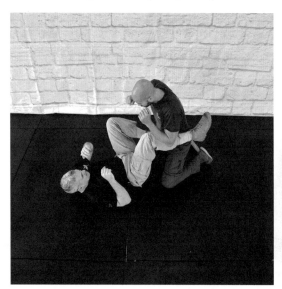 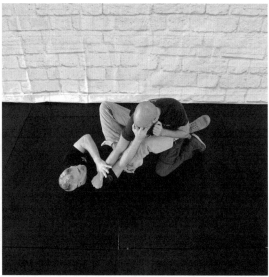

Foreleg brace into short triangle choke in defending a straight punch (single-attacker situation).

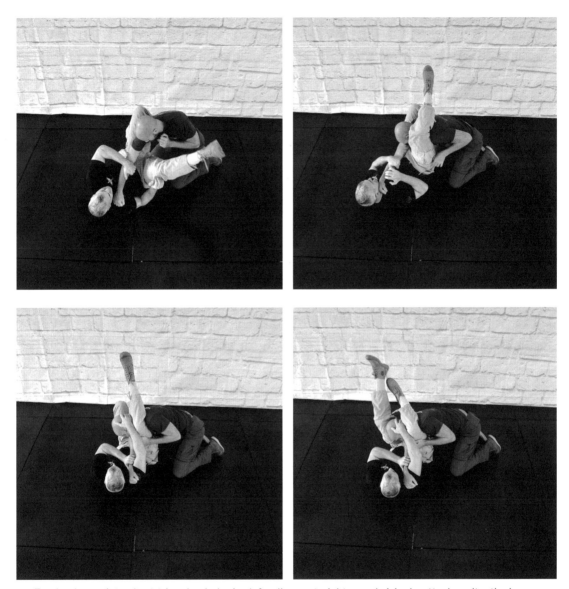

Foreleg brace into short triangle choke in defending a straight punch (single-attacker situation).

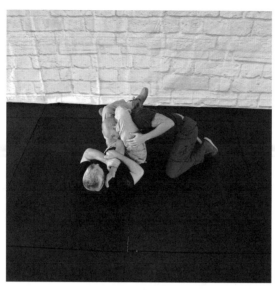

Foreleg brace into short triangle choke in defending a straight punch (single-attacker situation).

Forearm Short Triangle Choke

The forearm short triangle brace may be used if you cannot catch an opponent's arm to execute the previous leg triangle choke. The key, similar to the previous choke, is to trap the opponent's head between your legs. If you succeed in trapping his head only, you may then insert your own forearm underneath his neck to grasp your own ankle or pants leg. In the previous choke, you used the opponent's shoulder to place strong pressure on the underneath carotid artery, with your calf placing similar pressure on the topside carotid, restricting blood flow on both sides of his neck. This time you will use your radial bone. Squeeze your right leg down into his head while simultaneously clamping upward with your forearm. Pull the opponent's head into your torso to enhance the pressure. Be sure to turn slightly to create the optimum choking angle. **As always, be careful in training not to injure your partner.**

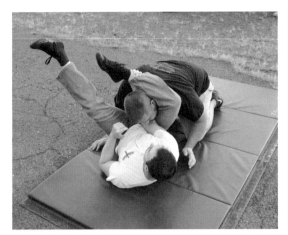 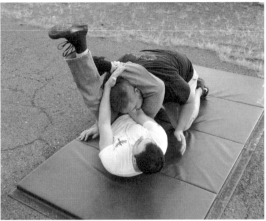

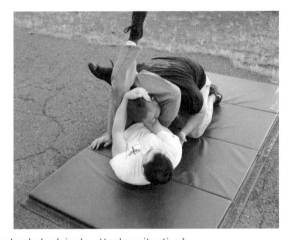

Forearm short triangle choke (single-attacker situation).

The descriptions given in the preceding combatives sections help you to learn when to use a technique and what to do—and what *not* to do—when you carry it out. Remember . . .

Correct Technique + Correct Execution = Maximum Effect

Index

Notable Biographies

Grandmaster Haim Gidon

Grandmaster Haim Gidon, tenth dan and Israeli Krav Maga Association president, heads the Israeli Krav Maga Association (Gidon system) from the IKMA's main training center in Netanya, Israel. Haim was a member of krav maga founder Imi Lichtenfeld's first training class in the early 1960s. Along with Imi and other top instructors, Haim Gidon cofounded the IKMA. In 1995 Imi nominated Haim as the top authority to grant first-dan krav maga black belts and up. Haim represented krav maga as the head of the system on the professional committee of Israel's National Sports Institute, Wingate. Grandmaster Gidon, whose professional expertise is in worldwide demand, has taught defensive tactics for the last thirty years to Israel's security and military agencies. Grandmaster Gidon is ably assisted by some of the highest-ranked and most capable krav maga instructors in the world, including Ohad Gidon (sixth dan), Noam Gidon (fifth dan), Yoav Krayn (fifth dan), Yigal Arbiv (fifth dan), Steve Moshe (fifth dan), and Aldema Zirinksi (fifth dan). More information is available at israelikrav.com and facebook.com/gidonsystemkravmaga.

Senior Instructor Rick Blitstein

Rick Blitstein is one of a few hand-picked individuals who traveled to Netanya, Israel, in 1981 to complete an intensive krav maga instructors' course. Under the watchful eye of krav maga founder Imi Lichtenfeld, Israeli experts taught Rick for the purpose of introducing krav maga to the United States. Imi and Rick formed a very close bond and spent much time training together in both Israel and the United States. For much of the past twenty years, Rick has worked in the field of private and corporate security, teaching and using krav maga in real-life situations. A member of the IKMA and recognized as a senior black-belt instructor, Rick is committed to the proper expansion of the system in the US and around the world. Rick sent the author to train with Grandmaster Gidon and the IKMA for advanced instructor certification. More information is available at israelikravmaga.com.

Kristof Sawicki

Kristof Sawicki is the IKMA chief instructor for Poland. He has an extensive background in martial arts, having begun his training in krav maga in 1995. He earned his black-belt degrees with Grandmaster Haim Gidon. Kristof has trained Poland's premier military units and has a large organization of schools throughout Poland. More information is available at www.krav-maga.pl.

About the Author

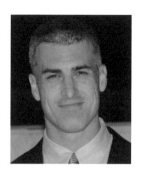

David Kahn, IKMA United States chief instructor, received his advanced black-belt teaching certifications from Grandmaster Haim Gidon and is the only American to sit on the IKMA Board of Directors. The United States Judo Association also awarded David a fifth-degree black belt in combat jiu-jitsu.

David has trained all branches of the US military; the Royal Marines; and hundreds of federal, state, and local law enforcement agencies. He has instructed at many respected military hand-to-hand combat schools, including the Naval Special Warfare Advanced Training Command (Imperial Beach), Marine Corps Martial Arts Center of Excellence (MACE Quantico), US Army Combatives School (Fort Benning), and at law enforcement academies including the FBI and DEA (Quantico), Philadelphia and New Jersey State Police, and a host of other academies.

David is also a certified instructor for the State of New Jersey Police Training Commission. He has created a modified krav maga football tactics program for marquee NFL and collegiate football players, including the 2017 and 2016 NFL Defensive Players of the year, Aaron Donald and Khalil Mack, Pro Bowler Olivier Vernon, and select players from the Jacksonville Jaguars.

David is regularly featured in major media outlets, including *New York Times*, *Men's Fitness*, *GQ*, *USA Today*, *Los Angeles Times*, *Washington Post*, *New Yorker*, *Penthouse*, *Fitness*, *Marine Corps News*, *Armed Forces Network*, *Special Operations Report*, and *Military .com*. He previously authored the books *Krav Maga*, *Advanced Krav Maga*, *Krav Maga Weapon Defenses*, *Krav Maga Professional Tactics*, and *Krav Maga Defense*.

David also produced the *Mastering Krav Maga* DVD series, Volumes I, II, III, and Volume IV Supplement: *Defending the 12 Most Common Unarmed Attacks*, along with the *Mastering Krav Maga Online* program. *Mastering Krav Maga Online* includes more than 500 lessons, amounting to more than forty-two hours of online study, covering approximately 95 percent of the krav maga civilian curriculum. For online training please visit masteringkravmaga.com. For additional krav maga information please see davidkahnkravmaga.com and facebook.com/davidkahnkravmaga.

David and his partners operate several Israeli krav maga training centers of excellence, along with the Israeli Krav Maga Advancement Program (IKMAP).

For more information visit israelikrav.com and davidkahnkravmaga.com.

US Headquarters:
Israeli Krav Maga US Main Training Center
860 Highway 206
Bordentown, New Jersey 08505
(609) 585-MAGA
israelikrav.com

Israeli Krav Maga Association (Gidon System)
POB 1103
Netanya, Israel
facebook.com/gidonsystemkravmaga

Training Resources
Asian World of Martial Arts
9400 Ashton Road
Philadelphia, Pennsylvania 19114
(800) 345-2962
awma.com

Aries Fight Gear
(800) 542-7437
punchingbag.com

Mancino Mats
1180 Church Road
Lansdale, Pennsylvania 19446
(800) 338-6287
mancinomats.com

BLUEGUNS®
Ring's Manufacturing
99 East Drive
Melbourne, Florida 32904
(321) 951-0407
blueguns.com

Authentic Israel Army Surplus
PO Box 31006
Tel Aviv 61310
Israel
US Local Phone: (718) 701-3955
Toll Free Number: (888) 293-1421
Israel: (972) 3-6204612; Fax: (972) 9-8859661
israelmilitary.com

To read more about krav maga and its history:

Israel Defense Force
Homepage: idf.il/en

Israeli Special Forces Krav Maga
Homepage: ct707.com

Israeli Krav Maga Association (Gidon System)
Homepage: israelikrav.com and facebook.com/gidonsystemkravmaga

BOOKS FROM YMAA

DVDS FROM YMAA

ADVANCED PRACTICAL CHIN NA IN-DEPTH
ANALYSIS OF SHAOLIN CHIN NA
ATTACK THE ATTACK
BAGUA FOR BEGINNERS 1
BAGUAZHANG: EMEI BAGUAZHANG
BEGINNER QIGONG FOR WOMEN 1
BEGINNER QIGONG FOR WOMEN 2
CHEN STYLE TAIJIQUAN
CHEN TAI CHI FOR BEGINNERS
CHIN NA IN-DEPTH COURSES 1—4
CHIN NA IN-DEPTH COURSES 5—8
CHIN NA IN-DEPTH COURSES 9—12
FACING VIOLENCE: 7 THINGS A MARTIAL ARTIST MUST KNOW
FIVE ANIMAL SPORTS
FIVE ELEMENTS ENERGY BALANCE
INFIGHTING
INTRODUCTION TO QI GONG FOR BEGINNERS
JOINT LOCKS
KNIFE DEFENSE: TRADITIONAL TECHNIQUES AGAINST A DAGGER
KUNG FU BODY CONDITIONING 1
KUNG FU BODY CONDITIONING 2
KUNG FU FOR KIDS
KUNG FU FOR TEENS
LIANG TAI CHI FOR HEALTH
LOGIC OF VIOLENCE
MERIDIAN QIGONG
NEIGONG FOR MARTIAL ARTS
NORTHERN SHAOLIN SWORD : SAN CAI JIAN, KUN WU JIAN, QI MEN JIAN
QI GONG 30-DAY CHALLENGE
QI GONG FOR ANXIETY
QI GONG FOR ARMS, WRISTS, AND HANDS
QI GONG FOR BETTER BREATHING
QI GONG FOR CANCER
QI GONG FOR ENERGY AND VITALITY
QI GONG FOR HEADACHES
QI GONG FOR HEALING
QI GONG FOR HEALTHY JOINTS
QI GONG FOR HIGH BLOOD PRESSURE
QIGONG FOR LONGEVITY
QI GONG FOR STRONG BONES
QI GONG FOR THE UPPER BACK AND NECK
QIGONG FOR BEGINNERS
QIGONG FOR WOMEN
QIGONG FOR WOMEN WITH DAISY LEE
QIGONG MASSAGE
QIGONG MINDFULNESS IN MOTION
QIGONG: 15 MINUTES TO HEALTH
SABER FUNDAMENTAL TRAINING
SAI TRAINING AND SEQUENCES
SANCHIN KATA: TRADITIONAL TRAINING FOR KARATE POWER
SCALING FORCE
SHAOLIN KUNG FU FUNDAMENTAL TRAINING: COURSES 1 & 2
SHAOLIN LONG FIST KUNG FU: ADVANCED SEQUENCES 1
SHAOLIN LONG FIST KUNG FU: ADVANCED SEQUENCES 2
SHAOLIN LONG FIST KUNG FU: BASIC SEQUENCES
SHAOLIN LONG FIST KUNG FU: INTERMEDIATE SEQUENCES

SHAOLIN SABER: BASIC SEQUENCES
SHAOLIN STAFF: BASIC SEQUENCES
SHAOLIN WHITE CRANE GONG FU BASIC TRAINING: COURSES 1 & 2
SHAOLIN WHITE CRANE GONG FU BASIC TRAINING: COURSES 3 & 4
SHUAI JIAO: KUNG FU WRESTLING
SIMPLE QIGONG EXERCISES FOR HEALTH
SIMPLE QIGONG EXERCISES FOR ARTHRITIS RELIEF
SIMPLE QIGONG EXERCISES FOR BACK PAIN RELIEF
SIMPLIFIED TAI CHI CHUAN: 24 & 48 POSTURES
SIMPLIFIED TAI CHI FOR BEGINNERS 48
SUNRISE TAI CHI
SUNSET TAI CHI
SWORD: FUNDAMENTAL TRAINING
TAEKWONDO KORYO POOMSAE
TAI CHI BALL QIGONG: COURSES 1 & 2
TAI CHI BALL QIGONG: COURSES 3 & 4
TAI CHI BALL WORKOUT FOR BEGINNERS
TAI CHI CHUAN CLASSICAL YANG STYLE
TAI CHI CONNECTIONS
TAI CHI ENERGY PATTERNS
TAI CHI FIGHTING SET
TAI CHI FIT: 24 FORM
TAI CHI FIT: FLOW
TAI CHI FIT: FUSION BAMBOO
TAI CHI FIT: FUSION FIRE
TAI CHI FIT: FUSION IRON
TAI CHI FIT IN PARADISE
TAI CHI FIT: OVER 50
TAI CHI FIT: STRENGTH
TAI CHI FIT: TO GO
TAI CHI FOR WOMEN
TAI CHI FUSION: FIRE
TAI CHI QIGONG
TAI CHI PUSHING HANDS: COURSES 1 & 2
TAI CHI PUSHING HANDS: COURSES 3 & 4
TAI CHI SWORD: CLASSICAL YANG STYLE
TAI CHI SWORD FOR BEGINNERS
TAI CHI SYMBOL: YIN YANG STICKING HANDS
TAIJI & SHAOLIN STAFF: FUNDAMENTAL TRAINING
TAIJI CHIN NA IN-DEPTH
TAIJI 37 POSTURES MARTIAL APPLICATIONS
TAIJI SABER CLASSICAL YANG STYLE
TAIJI WRESTLING
TRAINING FOR SUDDEN VIOLENCE
UNDERSTANDING QIGONG 1: WHAT IS QI? • HUMAN QI CIRCULATORY SYSTEM
UNDERSTANDING QIGONG 2: KEY POINTS • QIGONG BREATHING
UNDERSTANDING QIGONG 3: EMBRYONIC BREATHING
UNDERSTANDING QIGONG 4: FOUR SEASONS QIGONG
UNDERSTANDING QIGONG 5: SMALL CIRCULATION
UNDERSTANDING QIGONG 6: MARTIAL QIGONG BREATHING
WHITE CRANE HARD & SOFT QIGONG
WUDANG KUNG FU: FUNDAMENTAL TRAINING
WUDANG SWORD
WUDANG TAIJIQUAN
XINGYIQUAN
YANG TAI CHI FOR BEGINNERS

more products available from . . .
YMAA Publication Center, Inc. 楊氏東方文化出版中心
1-800-669-8892 • info@ymaa.com • www.ymaa.com